Never Giving Up on Myself

Angela H. Fitts

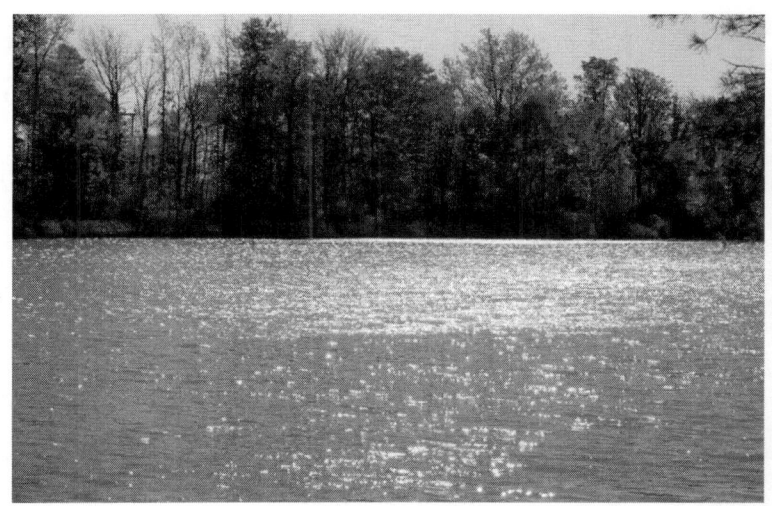

Never Giving Up on Myself
Copyright, 2022 by Angela H. Fitts

ISBN: 978-0-578-26629-9

Never Giving Up on Myself
Angela H. Fitts

Printed in Collierville, TN USA

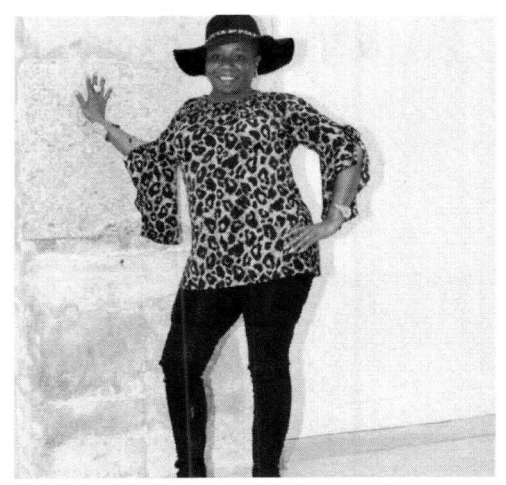

DEDICATION

This book is dedicated to my mother Gracy Lewis for believing in me. Thank you mom for holding my hands for 49 years. Thank you for cheering me on. I am so grateful to have your support. I want you to know you did an excellent job with me. I love you mother. I'm so proud to be your daughter.

To my stepfather Willie Lewis. Thank you for your prayers and support. Thank you for hearing my cry. You have taught me how to respect men. Thank you for believing in me.

To my boys Tevin Moten and Cortez Moten. I thank God for giving me three soldiers. I am grateful to be your mother. You all have made me a proud mom. I pray that you all continue to follow God and his word. I dedicated this book to you both. I change my life so that you both can be happy. I am so proud to have you both as my son. My two heart beats. To my daughter Nicole Moten. I have grown to love you unconditionally. I thank God for you. You have a sweet spirit that I admire. I am grateful to have you as my daughter.

To my brother Kevin Jordan, I am so proud to be your sister. You have made me proud. Thank you for being that brother I need. Thanks for loving me through my tough times. I will always love you.

To my oldest son Jeffrey Moten Jr. who is watching over me in heaven. I made history son. This is all for you. Rest in peace son.

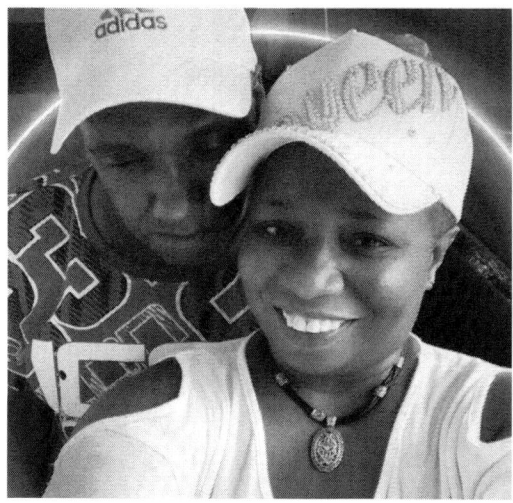

To My Husband

To my husband who held me down and never left my side. I wanted to thank you for loving me through my difficulties. I never knew marrying you would bring so much happiness in my life. You are the best deal I ever negotiated. Thanks for been my friend and lover. God is making a good wife out of me. I pray that our love will continue to grow. When I first said I do. I knew in my heart this will last forever. God has given me a king to love and cherish for the rest of my life. I know in my heart that choosing you was the best decision I made. I am honored to be your queen. Because of you. I believe I can fly!

Contents

Chapter 1

Hello, my name is Angela Fitts. I was born in Memphis Tennessee on September 27, 1972. I am a smart and outgoing person. I love to talk, sing, dance, and play music. Dancing is everything to me. Playing music keeps my mind at peace. I love being the Center of attention. I love to talk to people about their problems. I always wanted to be a leader. I knew what I wanted and went for it. I was a little shy in school. I was always to myself. What I did not like about myself, I did not speak up. I never stood up for myself when people who I care about do me wrong. I will react later. I enjoy going to school. I was a good student. I was quiet in school. My grades were fair. My conduct was outstanding. My attendance was perfect. I was outspoken and noticed. I always liked boys in school, but never approach them. I was tease by all my friends including the people I look up to. My friends will tease me for been skinny. After that I started to hate school. All my friends had developed faster than me. I did have good friends in school. One was Mary, she and I were close. We had the same issues; she also was extremely cute like I was. Mary and I spent the entire year best friends. Mary and I look out for each other. We talk on the phone all the time. Later, I did find out she slept with a guy that l was dating. I was shocked. They both hurt me. But it taught me not to trust a woman around your man. I had another friend in high school name Nancy, she stays in my neighborhood. She was very tall and dresses very well. She was different from other people. She had this attitude about herself. She did not let people get to her. We stay friends until they move from the neighborhood.

Nancy was a smart intelligent brave young woman. She was very neat and smart in school. Nancy and I share memories. I recall when her mom will invite us for dinner. This lady throws down in the kitchen. I remember Nancy and I will play school-teacher for the neighborhood. We will walk around and look for people to educate. We fed them and made sure they knew how to read and write. Nancy and I was close back then. I also want to share when I met my best friend, Yolanda. We attended the same church. We both went to Sunday school, bible class and sing in the choir. We all got baptize years ago, her and my brother, and her sister Karen. We all share great memories. Yolonda is like family. We were wearing ponytails when I met her. Yolonda and I have been friends over thirty years. I can go to Yolonda and talk to her about my problems without her judgement. Yolonda has always been a smart and independent woman. That is one thing we have in common. God kept our relationship together. Yolonda knows me inside and out.

She has been around when I had all three of my boys. We saw each other grow to be mothers and wife. I genuinely love her, and glad she was part of my life. Thank you Jesus for her.

When we were small, my mother will always take us to church every Sunday. We will be there before the sun comes up. This was every Sunday. We attended bible class on Wednesday night at 6 PM and followed by choir rehearsal. My mother was the President of the Usher Board. She taught Sunday school. She also was a speaker at church for years. She was good at talking to a crowd. I never knew how to do that. I was always afraid to. I was active in church. I always had a role in the church, just was afraid to speak out. I always saw my mom do it. I will always say that will never be me. My mother raised two kids, me and my brother Kelvin. I can say she did a great job as a single parent. My mom was an independent woman. I saw the struggle my mother went through with us. She did it all by herself and never gave up on us. I know I was a handful. I was hardheaded but I never disrespect my mother. I did things my mom was not pleased with. I am the oldest child. My mother never knew how to whip, but she did know how to put you on punishment. She will tell you no phone calls after 8 PM. We had to be in bed every night at 9 PM. No boys could not call me. Her rules were strong. One day she took the phone with her to work. So, I ask my friend Karen can I use her house phone. One morning, my mom call home. I had no ideal she would call. I answer the phone, it was my mother asking, why are you not at school. When my mother came home from work. She took the phone from me. I also did things like skip school. My mom found out. The school call my mother job, they usually call your house. This time they decided to call my Mother Job. I answer the phone thinking it was James. It was my mother asking, why are you not at school. I lied and told her I was not feeling well. Why didn't you call, she asks? She was mad and furious, told me to get my butt back to school. I was nervous because I knew I was in trouble with the school and my mother. Never got a chance to hear from my guy friend James. I went to school feeling afraid, of what the school was going to say or do. As I enter the school property, I saw police officers. In my mind, I thought the school have call the police on me for skipping school. I was full of fear. I decided not to go inside. The fear that ran through my body made me feel desperate. I call myself running away from home. I was only thirteen at that time. I ran to my best friend Trevika house. Trevika mom will ask me, do your mom knows you're here? I will lie and say yes. Trevika mom will ask questions I could not answer, because I did not have a plan. Later, she took me back home to my mother house. I had to tell the truth. I skip school to be with this guy name James Brown. He was my first narcissistic relationship. I met James through my friend Trevika. At a party in Clementine Apartments. It was in the summer. My first house party. There was so many guys and females at this party. I did have fun.

I had this other friend name Tonia. Tonia was a good girl. She loves gossip. Tonia and I had a lot in common, we love going to church. These two ladies, I will always talk to on a daily basic. We go back Elementary and Junior High. I looked up to them both. I felt like they were more advance than I was. Especially Trevika, she was driving, having sex, and having fun. I wanted to be around that. I met this guy name James. I hardly could not see him because the lights were off. He asks me for a dance. He asks can I see you again. I told him I did not know. I was 14. Trevika call me saying James like you. I said OKAY. I hardly knew this guy. He was older than me. I started talking to James on the telephone. He was a bad boy. People did not know that I like bad boys. Tonia and I will tell each other everything. I will talk to her about James. Tonia will talk about his friend Marvin. Marvin liked all of us. We did find that out later. Tonia looked up to Trevika more than she did me. I had a problem with that. She will get off the phone with me to talk with Trevika. I did not like that about them, but they still were my friends. I just wanted them to look up to me, not each other. I met up with James, when I visit Trevika in clementine. James will stare at me and smile. He gave me that look like I was his queen. I drove James's crazy when he saw me. I can sense it when he came around. When I start talking to James, I was head over hills in love. I went hard loving this guy. He was my first love. He was special to me in the beginning until he broke my heart. It did not take long for him to break my heart. He messes around and got some-one pregnant. James told me he wanted to be with her. That hurt my heart. This is my first time with a broken heart. I did not even tell Tonia about it at all. I knew I was not going to tell Trevika. She is the one who hook us up. She did not tell me he had another girlfriend besides me. She was friends with his girlfriend. Later I find out they became close friends. I felt betrayed by her and this guy she hooks me up with. She would never tell me things he does behind my back. She will tell Tonia about what he does. They will laugh about how he was cheating on me. Later, he come around like nothing happen, I accept him over and over. This heartbroken was so hard to carried. I knew I was wrong messing around with this boy, because I did not suppose be having sex or neither a boyfriend. I never mention to my mother about this guy name James. I know she will not have liked him. He did come over while she was at work. He will sneak over three times a week him and his friend. They will ride bikes all the way from Clementine to Airways Hood. James was one of the bad boys.

I always had a liken for the bad guys. I could not keep up with him, because my mom had these golden rules. She will tell my friends peaches cannot talk on the phone after 9 PM or she would say she cannot have phone calls from boys. They will make fun of me about that, especially Tonia. She always laughs because my mother was strict. So was her grandma. She had to sneak and do things to. We both were trying to be like Trevika because she was a beginner in everything we do. We wanted a piece of what she had going on in her life. Sex I had to pretend like I was having sex because I knew Trevika was. She ended up getting pregnant. I recall we went together for her to see was she. I was there with her the whole time. That is when I started bonding with her. I do not believe she liked me as a loyal friend. Later she ended up not been a friend of mine. She started hanging out with a different crowd.

Chapter 2

Meanwhile as time goes by, I am growing up a bit. Feeling myself. My little brother Kelvin was a sneaky person. What I mean about that mom thought he was a good boy. Little she knows he was mannish. He loves flirting with all my friends. I always had a problem with that. My brother did not like if his friends had a crush on me neither. Me and my brother was close growing up, I always looked out for him. We always stay into it as a child. I was always bossy with my brother. I knew, I will never do anything to harm him no matter how we fight or did not get alone. He was my only brother; I absolutely love him and his well-being. Me and my brother always had to share our things. We had to share and show love inside our home. My mom taught us to pray before we eat and go to bed. She taught me how to cook and sit like a young lady. I appreciate all what she shows me how to do. I know as a child I gave my mother a tough time. Yes, my mother always told me you weep what you sew. I heard that all through my childhood life. She also taught us to be responsible as kids. Not to open the door for strangers when she is not home. She also taught us to learn our phone number alone with knowing your social security number by hard. Date of birth your home address. We knew those things at the age of six. We had to learn these things because my mother had to work. I grew up fast, but my body development little slow. Mind you all my friends had butt's chest and hips. All I had was a little high butt.

People bullied me about that. One guy I hated so much me two years for been skinny. He would call me and my cousin Monica the bird family. Me and her was skinny coming up. I truly hated that about myself, made my self-esteem low.

My cousin and I grew up together. We did every-thing together. Monica and I share great memories growing up. What I love about my cousin she al-ways looks up to me. My brother loved playing sports in school. He was known at school. Like I mention early females were always into him. He thought he was the man back then. The girls made him feel like that when we were kids. My brother and I always protected our mother. I protected them both. We were close my mom and my brother. My mom raised us as a single parent. She was not married to neither one of our fathers. My father was not in my life period. He came around some-times. Not enough to build a relationship together. I did know who my dad was. I just never had a real relationship with him. I just learned that my father is narcissistic. Every man I ran across was just like him a narcissistic psychopath. My dad refuses to be in my life growing up, the first man that broke my heart was my dad. He always blames my mother for not been in my life. He never tries to get to know me as a person. That is when I start meeting guys just like him.

Later not knowing or having him as a father crippled my life toward been with a guy. I went out there looking for a man to love me. I never experience a man loving me the way a father supposed to love his child. I been around kids that had a dad at home. I just never had a dad at home. I also went out using my body looking for someone to love me. I never loved myself enough. I did later because pain taught me how to love myself. God plan was for me to not to know my dad. He saw something I did not see. Favor was in the mist not knowing who my dad was. I always worried about why my dad never try to get to know me. Just beating myself up.

I found out the hard way, let it go. I can author a book about absent parents in the home. How children suffer from it.

As time goes by, I met one of my brother's name Marquis. He is my half-brother on my dad side. I met him in the hospital. He was fighting for his life. I did get a chance to get to know him before he passes. Two full weeks. God meant for that to happen. The bound we shared before he left was something I will never forget. We both got a chance to share our pain. The pain we experience as a child. He heard my cry and I saw and felt his. I thank God for that two-week relationship we share together. I spent hours with him while he was fighting to live. I know in my heart he was grateful I was there with him. I did get a chance to meet his mother and his sister for whom he cared a great deal for. I continue to talk to his mother since he passes. What I did learned from my brother he was abandon just like

I was. He suffers in silent and ended up drinking. I also had another brother younger than me to. I can speak for me and both my brothers, not having you in our life did disturb us. I can say we had our mothers that play that role as a father. Melvin to you, God show me and both my brother's favor. Not having you in our life was the best thing for us. Lack of not having a father can affect us later. I read in the bible, I always had a heavenly father, who always loved me and never forsaken me. He was always there when I did not acknowledge him. Until this day. I decided to serve him and his people.

Meanwhile after dated this guy name James, I ran across another narcissistic name Eric Rogers. Never forget this guy. Eric was a different type of breed. He always made me laugh and smile. I met Eric through Karen. Met him in Walter Simmons

Apartments during the winter. He was a small skinny guy extremely easy to get alone with. I instantly took a liking to this guy. I introduced Eric to my mother because he was not a bad guy, and he also was not a good guy either. We will talk on the phone all night. I enjoy having sex with this guy all the time. We both had a crush on each other. My mother did like him in the beginning. She allowed him to go to the movies with us as a family. I cared a great deal for him until I got pregnant. That is when I found out how he was. He took off. I recall my mother calling his mother telling him my daughter is having a child by your son. His mom said he already has a kid; he does not take care of the child. His mother was letting my mother know, Eric is unfit to be a father. My mother was sad by all this, so was I. First time with a child. I was only about 14 no job, still in Junior High School. I was not older enough to have a baby. That is what my mother said. She at once took me to the doctor to have an abortion. After that I felt so empty and hurt for the third time. I just know I was a minor. The guy who got me pregnant was no good for me. He was a child himself. I was few months older than him. Later we lost connection with each other. I never heard from Eric Rogers again. As time went by, we moved by Airways School.

Meanwhile my mother gets a call saying her father died. That hurt me because he was my first role model. My grandfather was a very cruel man behind closed doors. At church, he would be this nice man with a fake smile. When he gets home, he takes his teeth out and be this other person. I never did understand his behaviors. During the summer, my mom will take us to the country, me and my brother. I always told my mother how I hated she left us there for weeks. I did enjoy going out there just to get away from Memphis. My grandfather always felt like I was a problematic child. He never complains about any of the grandkids. To him I was the outcast of the family. My granddad enjoys talking down on his kids when they were not around. I had to hear him say sad things about my mother and uncle Robert. When he sees them, he will not repeat what he had said bad about them. My grand mom was quiet. She kept to herself. She always did what my granddad said. I saw things she did for him, and I learned it applied it my life. Things I saw my granddad do I took in what I saw. Most things we saw in our family was wrong. I did learn things from my grandmother. My grandmom taught me how to shell black eye peas. I always watch her cook. I did learn how to press hair, and park. That was excited to learned. When my grand-dad died, she died on the inside. She truly shut down from the world and family. I never seen anything like it. Her spirit was gone as well. I hated that happen to her, because I never got that grandma love that you deeply needed from them both. I wish I could have done more for my grandma when she was living.

Meanwhile One sizzling summer I was getting my hair fix from my auntie Josephine. She was my first hairdresser. One day I caught the bus to my auntie shop to get my hair fix. She had this guy looking at her vehicle. This guy named Eddie Head showed me he was interested in me. Of course, I play hard to get because he was truly a different breed as well. He got my number from a source he says. He was years older than me not much. He was driving his own vehicle. He always carried a weapon. I always felt safe with this guy because he made me feel safe. We began to talk on the phone. Until he kept asking to see me. I finally decided to let him come through. I always fear this guy because he was a dangerous guy. He was always direct. My mother already knew of him. She just did not know we were talking. Brain was his real name. He loves driving me around showing me off. I truly felt safe with this guy because he will always tell me I will protect you. No one will never bother you if you with me. A man never told me anything like that period. Hearing something like that for the very first time made me want him even more. Eddie head also was a slim guy. A guy that likes to stay in trouble. From what I know about Eddie head he loves breaking the law. As I began to like him, I told my friends about him. He would pull up to my school with loud music. I was well known for how people look up to him. He would pick me up from school. He would always let the guys know that is my girl. I never had someone ride me around and appreciate the ground I walk on like he did. He would take me around my Ex James letting him know this my girl now. I enjoy it because James hurting me. So, making him jealous was on my

level. Eddie head was making sure when he is not
around people would respect his girl. At that time,
I thought that was cute. I learned the hard way that
was so toxic. He did that because he knew he had
an older woman and a baby that came with it.

One late Sunday night, he brought this girl to my
mom house. He called and told me he was coming
through. He asks my mom first can he come over.
When he did, he knock on the door ask for me. I
went outside thinking he had to ask me something.
As I went to the car, he had a lady in the front seat.
She got out the car told me get in. I got in sat in the
front with them. As I got in the car. I ask Eddie
head who was she. She said I am his lady. I was so
confused and bothered. Like why you would bring
your woman to my house. He said I wanted you to
know we got back together. I said you could have
told me this over the phone. She said "No," I told

him to tell you this in person. I was looking at them both as she was saying tell her the rest. I said there is more. She said yes. Did he tell you we have a child together? I said no, neither did he say he had a lady. He made sure I did not have anyone but did not mention he had a woman with a child. I said let me out the car, this is crazy! I do not need this. I remember him getting out the car tried to talk to me, as I try to go in the house. He was saying how he still loves me, but I have a family. I said to him please be with your family. I am still a minor. I am not advance like he was. I was afraid of his lifestyle. It was something like my first love James. Toxic, dangerous, and very abuse.

Chapter 3

I did learn a great deal dealing with the bad guys. They liked to abuse women, so I said let me find someone that goes to church. Here I am having my heart broken multiple times by different guys. I began to question myself, why I am getting dump by guys that already have females. All I know is it did not feel good. I started to feel insecure about myself. I started to think negative thoughts. Later those thoughts started to catch up with me. I truly gave my mother a tough time growing up. My mother always had these golden rules for the house. I had a tough time trying to do right by her rules. My mother was a little strict. She will sometimes listen to church members about how to raise me. My mother did not need their opinion on what to do with me. She already knew how to be a mother to me. Oh, I almost forgot to mention after we leave church. The Jordan family, we always did things together as a family. We will go to church then later stay down my granddad house all my siblings, cousins, aunties, uncles. We will have the time of our life. Playing kick ball as a family, eating dinner, laughing, and talking. The whole Jordan family. I will never forget those moments. The Jordan family still gets together on Thanksgiving and Christmas. We always had an enjoyable time back in the days. I remember as a child we had fun together. How we all laugh and dance. I deeply miss those days. That was when Jordan family was close. We are not like we should be. I know we still loved each other as a family. The Jordan Family Rocks. I just wish we can be like we use to be. As time goes by, I started to go to Airways Jr. High School. I was happy when we move in a new neighborhood. Moving was like a new beginning. I felt like this is going to be a fresh start for me. We move in a nice house. My mother manages her business as a mom. I learned how to do just that. I learned quick from my mother. She taught me how to pay bills and how to cook and sit like a lady. She always talks to me about boys. We always had that mother and daughter talk. Later she ended up putting me on birth control.

While living in my new neighborhood I met so many people. I felt known when I first move there. So many guys were spending time together in the neighborhood. The females I met was all cool to be around. I had this friend name Karen who stay in the neighborhood and Chandra. They both were a little younger than me. These girls were having fun and during big girl stuff. I had to sneak to do that. I try to act like I do these things so I can fit in. I also had friends in the neighborhood, his name is Mario Haywood. He was the only friend that I cared about. I can depend on him when I was sad or needed someone to talk to. Things start to change when he went to jail. Mario was a great friend, we stayed connected through letters and phone calls. I always stood by his side. I also met Mario family. They stay in the code by Gary's Super Market. He had two sisters. One who I became close friends with. I call her pudding. Her real name is Taurus. She was very shy back then when I met her. She was carrying a child when I first met her. I did like her when I met her, but I continue been friends with her brother. As of today, pudding and I remain friends. I saw her grow as a woman to a queen. Now she owns her own business. I do show her support. I love pudding with all my heart. She is one of my loyal friends I will never forget, and I will always keep her close to my heart.

One Summer evening, me and my brother Kelvin decided to go to the store. I was in a good mood this day. Looking good feeling good about myself. We walk down this street call bird. I do remember seeing certain people I knew. Through the crowd comes this guy named Patrick. He was short with a small afro and curly hair, chubby too. He walks up to me saying you look good. He had this look in his eyes that he saw something in me. I told him I had a man. He repeated what I said. I told him my brother was my man. So, I went inside the store. When me and my brother came out the store, there he was standing around outside the store. I did not say anything to him, but he did walk up to us saying your lady looks good. He even walks us home so he can know where I stayed. He also gave my brother a pager so he can keep up with me. I just know he was moving fast. He would always ride down my street hoping he would see me outside. He would sometimes take me and my friends to school. He also would take all of us out to eat. Showing off his charm and money, so he can get what he wants from us. We will always try to jump out the car so none of us would end up in the car with him. All my friends thought like Patrick was creepy and strange. He was very controlling could not take no for an answer. What I did like about Patrick is he had a vehicle and he was a smart guy, very dependent. What I did not like, he will use his money to control women.

As time went by, Patrick will sometimes pick me up from work. I was 16, working at Wendy's and going to school. I recall he would always be on time to pick me up. Patrick would always flirt with people I know. I will always address him about it. He never liked for me to question him about his action. This was one of the red flags I should not have ignored. I did know he liked me. One night I call him to pick me up from work. This night I was truly tired. I normally would have asked my mom to get me, but I knew she was tired from working. Plus, it was after 10:30 PM. She had to be back at work in the morning. Patrick picks me up that night. He waited in the parking lot for me to get off. As I got into his vehicle, he asked me to ride with him to his apartment. I said where? He never would say. I did tell him I have to be home before 12. He continues to ignore the rules my mom gave me. All he said was you acting like a little girl. I felt like I was not a little girl. I just did not want to be push. Plus, he was older than me, I did not want him to continue calling me a little girl. So, I let him talk me into going where he wanted me to go. As we were going into the apartment complex, I truly got nervous. As we got out the car to enter the door. He asked me was I ready. I look into his eyes and say ready for what? I did notice there was no furniture inside as we walk toward the bedroom. I told him while he was laying on the bed, I got to be home. He did not care. I said to him I was ready to go home. He said to me go ahead and leave. I look at him and said are you serious. I needed for him to take me home. I had no clue where I was, he noticed I felt out of place. He shouted out to me go and leave. I felt so trap. I did not have a cellar phone back then, only pager. They had pay phones back then. I ask him can I use his bathroom. I went to the bathroom and started to cry because I was in a situation. I did not want to have sex with him not on that night anyway. While I sat in there taken my time, he was saying hurry up stop acted like you a virgin. You knew what this was going to be like. Truly I did not. I just was not ready. I finally came out the restroom sat on the end of the bed. He asked me to take my jacket off get comfortable. Telling me you are safe with me. I remember him trying to kiss me. I rejected him. I noticed that made him snap at me. He screamed out I was a little girl. I need a woman not a child, do not call me anymore. Then he said to me why are you here if you cannot do what I say. I tried to tell him I was not ready. He kept on pushing his self on me. Fussing and shouting in my ear, you do not act right you will walk home. I close my eyes. I let him do what he wanted to do with my body. I told this guy; I was on my cycle. He did not care. He climbs on top of me and raped me. I cry the whole time. He belittles me as he noticed me in tears. He continues to rape me knowing I was saying stop please stop. He would get more aggressive with me. He tried to treat me harsh while having sex with me. Told me I do not deal with little girls. You are crying like I am hurting you. Then he said you knew what this was going to be like. I went to the bathroom crying to myself. Ready to go home hoping this night will be over. I cry out to God that night. He also did not use protection at all. I told him while he had taken me home, he raped me. He got mad start calling me names because he knew that will make me cry. I never felt so degraded in my entire life. He took advantage of my body. Made me feel like a cheap prostitute. I never felt like this with any guy I been with until I met him. This was the beginning of hell for me. When he took me home, I did not say any-thing to nobody. Did not want to hear from this guy ever again. I wanted to tell someone so bad what I experienced. I was screaming in the dark. I was thinking it was all my fault this happen to me. He made me feel like I deserve it. I stayed in the house a month.

Later I ran across him after he tried to call and stalk my house. Did not want to run across him. I was ashamed in so many ways. I never experienced something so ugly and devastated. I truly tried to stay hidden so he could not find me. When I did finally see him, He was someone else. Talking to me like he did not know he took control of my body. Rape me while I was on my cycle. When I brought it up to him, he tried to brush it off. He truly ignored me at all costs. When I kept throwing it up, he flips out. It did not take long for that mask to slip. This time I was able to walk away because I was close to my house. He followed me home saying he did not mean to do that. Blaming me for his behavior. I started letting him sucker me up with his Bull. As time went by, I start caring for this guy. He always was around me in the beginning. Patrick always did everything I needed him to do in the beginning. He hardly talks, I was always the one who did the talking. When I met him, he was 18? I was sweet 16 hitting 17. The minute I start telling him I love him; he shows me who he really is. I really thought he was the one. He came by my house with this girl in the car name Brenda. I already knew who she was. She was laughing saying come go with us. Repeated it over and over. I decided to go because I wanted to know who this lady was with Patrick. They pull up to my mom house with the loud music. I went to the car. Big Charles was driving while Patrick and Brenda rode in the back seat together. I got in the front seat. While riding away from my house. I hear Brenda yelling and laughing stop Patrick. Repeated it over and over. The feeling I had going through my body felt like pure trauma. Something you will never want to experience. He knew this was hurting me, but he did not care. I was trying my best not to cry. I remember Charles asking me was I OK. I could not moment a word. Patrick decided we were going to go to the Skating Ring. Patrick pays all our way to get in. He had to show off like he always does. Me and Brenda was talking while Patrick was feeling like he was the man. I hardly knew her. I just know we both liked him. Patrick would do things like that to make me jealous. After we left the skating ring, we all headed home. I remember Patrick telling Charles to drop peaches off at the house. Me and Brenda going out to have fun. That hurts me hearing Patrick saying this aloud. I started to hate myself because I allowed this man to treat me like this. I felt so low! I started to lose myself in all of this. When he drops me off? I decided not to go home. I went over my friend house name Karen. I knew she would be up. I did not tell her anything about what I experience with Patrick. Karen felt like I can do better. I did not talk about Patrick to any of my friends, because I saw him flirt with them in my face. Later, I spoke with Brenda the next day. She was crying on the phone. I asked her what was wrong. She screamed out Patrick rape her. I could not say a word. I felt so bad because here I am pregnant by this guy. I did believe her because he did me to. I listen to her spill the tea on Patrick. After all that I still end up with him. I never heard from Brenda at all since then. She was one of the women's that truly got away. I did know she had dated him before me. Later I mentioned it to Patrick what Brenda said to me, he went into a rage and said harsh words. I never mentioned her again.

Chapter 4

As time went by, I attended Melrose High School. Patrick was jealous of everything I do. Back then I thought that was cute. He must love me. He got even worst with his jealous and insecurities. He would confuse me with the rules my mother made for me. I would always remind him I cannot be out late or do all the things he wanted me to do. He would bully me by saying, you are a little girl. Listen to your mom because I need a woman to do what I say. He also will say I can take care of you. Later I started to disobey my mother rules by sneaky out the house. Climbing out the window so I can be with Patrick. I knew what I was during was wrong. I knew it will be a wrap if my mom caught me. My little brain thinking, Patrick got me like he said. I also would sneak Patrick in my mother house. I would sneak him through the window. He would stay hours. Then later he started staying all night. He did not want to go home. He knew I was afraid to do this. I could not sleep at all when he made me do these things. I felt so unsure. I was always trying to prove myself to this guy ever since I met him. I lost myself in this. One time I did something wrong that caused me to run away from home and move in with Patrick and his mother. I thought this would be a good thing to do. He was excited that I did this. He would take me to school every morning. I felt out of place standing with Patrick and his family. The feeling was intense. My heart would not allow me to enjoy my freedom. I felt bad on top of it. I began to hate where I was. Patrick started having rules for me as well. He did not want me to join activities at school. He did not want me to be a cheerleader. He will always pick me up on time from school. He would be mad if it took me a long time to come out the school building. He will fuss at me for insignificant things. Like whom you were talking to at school. Do not wear lip stick. My girl does not talk back. He was so controlling. I also got into trouble at his mom house that police had to be call. The officer asked me for ID. The officer said we have a call on you for running away. So, they took me to juvenile. I stay there overnight. Meanwhile the officer calls my name and said time to go home. I am thinking my mother got me out. Patrick got someone to play like they were my mother. They were able to pull it off. I did not plain this at all. I was happy to see him. The other side was afraid as well. I still was considering a runaway because, my mother found out later who got me out. She had to report it again. The officer came back over to pick me up from Patrick's mother house. They took me back to juvenile until my mother got me out. I knew what I did was wrong. I knew better. I just wanted to fit in. I wanted to please a man that I thought was the world to me. I did terrible things just to be with this monster. I disobeyed my mother, broke the law and rules for him. My mother always says karma is something else. You weep what you sow my mother will always say. I did not think so much of it until I start having kids by this monster.

Living with Patrick and his mother was pure hell. His sisters stay there so did his brothers. They could have people come over all night and play-house. His mother made it comfortable for me to live there. Gave me and Patrick a room upstairs. I know my mother would not allow that at her house at all. I saw Patrick flirting with females in front of me while living with his family. He would try to disrespect me in front of his family. I will always stand up for myself. He did not like for me to cuss at him like he does me. He tried his best to train me to obey him or shut the hell up while he is talking.

He also wanted me to sit around while he does his cheating. I will always question him about him sleeping around with other females. He was a big liar. Everybody in the community had him. Later I found out I was with child. Yes, Patrick was excited about it too. A way that he can tied me down. I thought when I became with child, he will change, and he will treat me better. Maybe show respect because we are having a child. He treated me like garbage. I never told a soul how he treated me. He gave me this ring and said we were married. He also said he did not want anyone to tell him different. I would repeat to him what my mother said about us not been married. He will go into a rage about what she said. He felt like he did not need anybody to say he is married. He wanted that power and control. He did not listen to me about the rules he made for me. He will make sure I stay away from family and friends. Anyone that can influence me about him. He would keep them away from me. I would listen to him. Whatever he said goes. I did it because; I fail in love with him. I could not think. He thought for me. I lost myself. He was my God. I put this man before God and myself. As I carried my first child. I experienced so much pain with this man. He did not take me to no doctor appointments at all. Now he has me walking to school. In the beginning, he had taken me everywhere I needed to be. I was so depressed. I felt bad that I was pregnant by Patrick. He would cheat right in front of me. He would start to ride down my street with different women to make me jealous. It truly made me more stressful. My body started to change. Here I am underage having a baby. Still living with my mother in high school. I had so many things going across my mind. I cry all while I was with child. I remember he went to jail for months in another state. He was riding around with drugs in the car. He stays in jail for over three months. When he got lock up, he would call my mother house collect. I would accept those calls. He told me not to worried I will pay for those calls. Yes, he paid for it, after my mother brought it to his attention. He honestly thought that would control my mother. Later, I ended up having my first born. Patrick Moten Jr. August 28, 1990, at 2 AM six pounds and nine ounces. I ended up having a handsome baby Boy. That was one of the happiness days of my life. My mother and Auntie Jeanette was there when I had Patrick. They stay there to the end. I was truly afraid. I could not do it without their help and support. Patrick was not around when I had my baby. I really do not remember where he was at that time. I was still living with my mother when I had my first born. My mother taught me how to be responsible. I learned quick. Having a child will change you and grow you up. I had to continue to work. I had to help my mom pay bills. I was having trouble during that because I had a baby. I did not have transportation to get around.

That there was hard all by itself. She will always remind me you made this child, your responsibility. I learned that fast.

Later, my mother took me and my son to live with my auntie. We helped each other out. She had three kids and I had only one. My auntie Jeanette always worked two jobs. She was a single woman tried to take care of herself and her kids. I was crazy about my auntie kids. She had one girl name Tiffany and a son name Mario Jordan and Antonio. While living with My auntie we became close we look out for one another. She was more than just my auntie she was a sister a friend and a mother to all my boys. I also let Patrick stay with us as well. He would take my auntie to work. He came in and took control of everything. He was a handy man. He slept around with my Auntie. I did not find out until later. I do not know how long this has been going on. The signs were there. I just did not want to believe she would do this. I never question neither one of them about it. Me and my auntie stop talking for a long time about this. Well, I stop talking to her. I do not know if she was aware why. My heart tells me she does know. I do know they hardly could not get alone. She would bash him in front of family. He would call her out her name behind closed doors like he did me. I always wonder why he would talk to my auntie like that. Later is when I put it all together how narcissistic are. They care less who they hurt or sleep around with. They have no boundaries at all. They also do not protect themselves while having sex. They will lie to you day after day. They will also ghost you for weeks, months, sometimes a year. They always have another victim on the side.

Later I moved out my auntie house stay with my narcissistic dad. The worst mistake I made was moving in with him. I wanted to call my mom and tell her I am so sorry. I never did. My ego got the best of me. I knew my mother did not want Patrick around her house. While living with my dad he also said Patrick could not come over there or stay all night. He made sense. My dad did not like Patrick hanging around if it did not help him. He liked him in the beginning because they both were getting something out of it. Them both been narcissistic finally play out. Patrick did not move us into a place at all. My dad really did not want me living with him. So, he went on and let me and my first born lived with him. My dad was a diligent worker. He went to work every day. Kept his house clean and neat. My dad was on drugs. He will steal my money, and later he will put it back in there. He did not think I knew. When I started hiding my money, he got very ugly. I mentioned to him I saw him getting my money. Things went left from there. I wanted so bad to find me a place to stay. My dad would always complain about my son been on his bed. It really was a tight spot to be living with him. I was stepping on eggshells living with my dad Melvin. One day I went looking for me a place to stay. I never told anyone that I was moving. I remember staying with Pudding for a week before I move in my place. I was hiding from Patrick and my dad. My son was with his family on his dad side. I needed time for myself. I did not tell Pudding what I was going through at all. I was screaming on the inside for help. Pudding opens her home for me. All I did was sleep because I was so depressed. Pudding was married with a family. I knew pudding had enough going on in her life. So, I left pudding house going back to my dad house ready to move. The day I was moving, me and my dad got into a fight. One day he came home early, while I was in the middle of getting my things together. He came home in a bad mood. He went into his bed-room. He saw my son on his bed. He snaped again. He said why is your son on my white sheets. He is getting it dirty get him off. Talking like my son was a stranger to him. He treated us like we were his slaves. As he was screaming about my baby on his bed. Meanwhile I was in the middle of packing, Melvin came toward me asking, where you are going. Saying I am always up and down the streets. Shouting all in my ear in a rage. He grabbed my bag as I was packing. He poured my clothes out the bag. When my clothes hit the ground, his towels fail out. That is when the mask slip. He grabbed me by my neck said your stealing my towels. He slammed me in the wall. Left a big hole in it. Now I am Thinking like this must be normal, because now my dad is hitting on me. I felt like I deserve it. I cried for months. I left his house on a bus. I never looked back.

Chapter 5

I already had the key to my own place. I just did not have any furniture. I did not call my kids father at all. I did not want to be around any man at all. I knew this was something I had to do alone. I did just that, I escape. I am now living in my own place. Me and my only son Patrick. I got settle in my new place. Got myself modern furniture for my home. I caught the bus to work. I also put my son in a day care so I can be able to work. Things started to get better for me and my son Patrick. I decided to contact my mother. My mother helps me get modern furniture for my place.

As time goes by, now that I am on my feet here comes Patrick. He will disappear at times. He would go and lived with other females. I got immune to his behavior. I let this clown back into my life. Thinking he would do right by me and his son, not at all. He got me pregnant for the second time. I still had my job, while I was with child. I still had to take care of the bills and my son Patrick. Plus, I had a child on the way. Patrick was still messing around with different females. He made life hard for me. He would take me to work, but he would not pick me up. He did this so many times. There will be time he will not show up. I had to catch two busses to get home. Then try to make it home to get my son off the day care bus. I recalled how Patrick will pick on me just because I was happy. He was so jealous of me and my son. He hated to see me giving Patrick attention. He was so cruel and selfish. I finally end up having my son Tevin. He was born at 2:30 AM that morning, eight pounds and two ounces. I remember having him like it was yesterday. His dad was not around when I had him.

I call his twin sister to take me to the emergency hospital. They both rushed me there. One of his twin sisters named my son Tevin. Having Tevin made my world complete. Tevin made me smile as a mother, he was always trying to prove himself. Tevin always was a Mama's boy. I had to learned fast, how to make ends meet. The struggle was real been a single parent with two. I never gave up. Meanwhile, Patrick refused to help me with the boys. He was so busy running behind the females. Patrick got this other lady named Stephanie pregnant. Her daughter was the same age my son was. She called me telling me Patrick was cheating on me with her. Later he ended up going to jail. When he returned to jail, he will be this perfect guy. He will help me with the bills and show how grateful he is.

One summer I was at work, I get a visit from Stephanie. She came up there to let me see her daughter.

As she approached me with her child. She introduced herself to me. She said hi I am Stephanie, Patrick baby Mom. I spoke with you on the phone. I remember talking to her on the phone. She did mention to me she wanted me to meet her daughter. I just never thought like I should. As I was looking at her daughter, Stephanie was asking me do she looks like Patrick. My heart drops, my blood was boiling hot. I did not have words for this lady. She did not know how that made me feel coming up to my job, thinking I needed to see her daughter. I was not ready for all that. I tried to play it cool as she shows me her daughter. I always wondered why she felt like she needed to do that. I knew she was crazy about him just Like I was. After she left my job. I had to go home. I was not able to stay at work. Here I am going through another type of pain. These pains came in levels. They all felt horrible. When I got home, I waited for him to call me. He was lock up at that time. Our kids were weeks apart.

He was busy screwing the community. When he finally called me. I told him how I hated him, he was furious. He could not get a word in. He knew I was mad. So, I stopped visiting him in jail, stopped answering his phone calls. Few weeks later, he had his vehicle pull from my house. I woke up one Sunny Morning headed to work. I put my boys on the day care bus, I noticed my car was gone. I call in letting the job know I could not come to work. That is when he got my attention. He knew just what to do. I was back in his present again, doing everything he ask me to do.

When he got out of jail, we continued to argue and fight. I recalled him doing this in front of the boys. He will pick a fight with me so he can see other women. He always will rape me after he jumps on me. He enjoyed seeing me crying while having sex with me. I did not feel any love from it. I hated how he treated me. He shown me his true color. As time went by, I was having his third child. I kept myself a job so I can survive for my boys. When I had his last child. We were on bad terms. He would always jump on me while I am caring his child. You would think this guy would not hit a woman with a child. Those other two times I was with child, Patrick was in jail. This last child I had he was around. He treated me poor. I cried while he was around. He degraded me as a mother and girlfriend. One night I beep him 911, he knew that means I am having a baby. He came through when I text 911. That night it was very cold outside. He ran into my house yelling wear their clothes at. Hurry up I got to go. He was saying come on to our boys. I was ready to go, he looks at me and said you are not going. I saw the look he had in his eyes. He said, I came to get the boys call 911. You good at calling them on me. As he was walking out the door, I look out the door. I saw a female getting out the car helping my other two boys get into the car. I call out to him as I was walking toward the car in pain. My body was in mission to have his baby. He pulled off so fast as he knew I was walking toward his car. I felt so abandon after he did that to me. I sat there in pain crying hoping he would come back. He never did. I wanted to die at that moment. I felt like nobody loves me. I was so afraid to call my mother about this. I needed her so bad. I just did not want her to know how bad he had treated me. I wanted her to think that everything was okay, when really, I was screaming for help. I ended up calling my brother Kelvin to take me to the hospital. I explain to him what was going on. He at once came. I had my last baby January 5, 1995, at 1:45 AM. He was seven pounds and two ounces. He made me a proud mom. I was in so much pain and hurt. My blood pressure was not at all normal. He truly brought happiness back into my life. Later Patrick came to the hospital to see me and his son. He came with one of his friends, Deon was his name. He also had that same woman from last night. He was holding our baby when I got a phone call. The lady on the phone said tell Patrick if he does not hurry up, she will set it off. I got my son from him told him to please leave. He knew I was furious. He did not give a dam. He truly was having a thrill seeing me hurt. He truly was getting a hard on from it. When I noticed it. I saw how sick this man really is. He truly was in my life to kill, steal, and destroy me. When it was time for me to go home from the hospital. He refused to pick us up from the hospital. I finally found me a way home with our newborn.

When I got home my lights were off. Patrick promised me he would pay the light bill, which was all he had to do. Until I get back on my feet from having his baby. While I am at home settle down with his baby. I call him screaming at him about the lights, he came over. Looking like he so concern. Did not pick us up from the hospital at all. I was so mad at myself. I said to myself, why do you continue calling this guy to help you. I end up staying with his mother for two weeks. I cried the whole time. His mother saw the hurt in me. He even had his females come over asking to see his baby. I did not know what he was telling them, but from the look of it. He tells them, she just my baby mom. He also fools them just like he did me! We all had our equal share with this monster. I ended up going back to work when my son was three weeks old. I had to because living with his mother and family was not for me. I been down that road living with the family. I borrowed money to get my lights cut back on. Patrick had the money; he just refuses to help. Later I got my bills caught up. Finally, I got my taxes and pay cash for me a new car. I finally decided to move out and find me and my boys a bigger place to stay. I was making things happen.

Having three boys brought so much joy into my life. I thank God for my three boys. That is the best thing, I got out this relationship was my three Heart Beats. He could not take that happiness away when he was present. He was jealous of the attention me and my boys share with one another. From what I gather, he never got that as a child. He never knew how to share love with any of his kids. Neither did he know how to love a human being. Me and my kids was living our best life without his help. He ended up in jail again. I had to make ends meet. I had to make sure I keep my car support and my bills caught up. I had a good paying job that kept me out of other people pocket. I will continue to talk to Patrick over the phone. I always made sure he stays in his boy's life. I never kept them from their dad.

Meanwhile I continue to support myself and kids. I end up running into one of my friends in school. Her name was Nancy. She stays with me for over five months. She moves in with me because she had no place to stay. We ended up helping one another. She had a son that she had with her. Mind you she did not have a car or a job, no income at all. I helped her because we were best friend years ago. She kept my house clean and always cook dinner. I was always working long hours, while she took care of the house. She did an excellent job in the beginning. She also found a job dancing. She would come home drunk with different guys. Things started to make a U turn when she started getting money. She would have different guys at my home, while I was at work. I try to tell her how I feel about all these guys coming through. She would act a fool about it. She had people thinking it was her place. Nancy will steal my car and go pick up guys knowing I had to work. There will be times she will not come home. I was stuck with her son. She would come to my job and get him. I got so tired of her bull, I told her she had two weeks to find her somewhere to stay. She started acting a fool. Told me she was not going anywhere. She wanted to talk crazy So, I ended up telling her she had to leave now. She wanted to fight. Telling me I owe her money. I call the police on her to escort her out my house. Two days later she bust my windows out my house, and flat my tires on my car. What a bad choice she did. I wanted to kick her ass. Instead, I got her locked up. I had no time to be going to jail fighting a woman that had nothing to lose. I had boys that needed their mother on a daily basic.

After getting rid of another headache. I met this guy name Mark. Mark was younger than me. He had brown eyes that always change to green. He was a handsome guy that truly was crazy about all my boys. He would always get them off the bus when I was running late from work. He really did not have to. He did it because he cares about us. I did not like him in the beginning, to me he was like a handy man around the house. He never tried to come on to me at all. He would always come over and play the game with my boys all day. I will always make sure he is fed. Later we became good friends. I knew I can trust him. I was still talking to Patrick while he was in jail. Later I start picking up habits, I was going to clubs, taken myself on adventure, going on Beale Street. Patrick kept those things from me. He did not want to see me happy. I was able to do what I wanted to. I was trap been in a relationship with Patrick. Mark was hanging around daily. One night I was drinking with Mark. I decided to ask him did he like me. Of course, he said Yes. I asked him what he was willing to do to be with me. He said anything you want or ask of me. Never heard a man say that at all. I can tell he was nervous. Mark fail head over hills with me. Now we are living together. Later Patrick heard about Mark. Nancy told him all about Mark. She always did sneaky stuff behind my back. Mark knew about my kid's father. He would call me collect while Mark was there. In the beginning Mark was okay with it. When Mark started having feelings, he wanted to tell me what he did not like. I was not trying to hear it. I felt like I am in my own spot, and I do not need rules. I told Mark you knew what you were getting yourself into. Mark wanted me to stop accepting his collect calls. I told Mark "No," which is not happening.

Chapter 6

Finally, Patrick got out of jail. Mark was living with me. I did not want to kick Mark out at all. He was helpful to me, plus I liked him. Later Patrick started calling me saying he wanted to see the boys. I said OKAY. I thought like Patrick was coming over to pick them up. Not at all, he came in and sat down on the couch. It was like walking on eggshells, having my kids' father over and Mark pacing the floor. I did not like this at all. Patrick was enjoying this; it is like he did this before. I did not know how to tell Patrick to leave. I was having my first anxiety attack. Patrick did this on purpose. Mark was already drinking, so he let his alcohol get the best of him. Patrick would start coming over when he got ready. I really did not want Patrick back. One night me and Mark were drinking and Patrick pop over, acting like he wanted to see his kids. They were asleep. I went to the door there was Patrick at the door, looking like someone has broken his heart. Patrick asked me, where my boys. I said they are asleep. He walked in and sat on the couch, asking me to wake them up. Mark came from the back mad, I was trying my best to keep peace. I knew I had to make rules for them both. I had to remind them both this is my house. I went into the bedroom, while Patrick was playing with one of the boys. Mark and I were arguing about Patrick been at my house. Mark was holding me down on the bed, trying to make me listen. I did not want to hear none of it. I just wanted peace in my home. Patrick heard me and Mark in the room. He ran into the room and jumps Mark. I did not like what was going on. Patrick knew he was out of place. He already had a woman. Meanwhile, I left my home and came back later. Only person who was there was Mark. Patrick left with the kids.

When I got back home. Mark was crying, thinking I left him to be with Patrick. I knew then it would be hard to get rid of Mark. At this point, I just wanted out. I was dealing with two psychopaths at the same time. I tried to talk to Mark about what I was going through with him and Patrick. He was not hearing it. All he kept saying was please do not leave me, I love you. Mark began to start drinking in the mornings without eating breakfast. He started missing work to see if I was with Patrick. I started feeling isolated with him. Both guys were driving me insane. I decided to break up with Mark and told him, I needed time. He started crying saying he loves me and the kids. I went into a depression mood. Here I am working 12-hour job, making good money. I truly did not need anybody in my way. I was becoming an independent woman.

Meanwhile, the apartment I was living in needed to be fixed. I was always working never had time. I was working a 12-hour shift. I could not take a day off from work. The job requires for us to be at work every day. One day my car broke down. That hit the fan. I did not ask anyone to take me to work. I started thinking negative about everything. I started drinking, to keep my mind off my problems. I had all three of my boys at home with me. I had a week to be out my apartment, I just was not prepared. I did not even know how to go to God. Neither did I think to reach out to my mother. I was complete alone in the dark hurting. I truly was asking God to take my life. I felt like a failure at this time. I cried the whole night. I did not have anybody to babysit my boys. I remember calling Yolanda after 11 PM. She answers the phone. She knew something was wrong. I was telling her; I did not want to live. She was trying to talk to me, I end up passing out. The next thing I know the

73

ambulance was at my house. Yolonda came through for me. I took aspirin while I was drinking alcohol. I remember crying out to Yolanda about my problems. I start throwing up, while she was on the phone. I lost control and hit my head. When I woke up, I was at the Med. When I realize what was going on. I explain to them about my car breaking down. They were telling me you are going to be fine. We will let your job know, where you are. I also explain to them, I must find me a place to stay. They wrote my information down. Asking me questions about my job and were I lived. I explain to them the best I could. They gave me something to calm me down and told me everything will be okay. I did not tell them about my mother, because I was mad at her for the things I was going through. She never told me that love will hurt. I was afraid to share with her, what I was going through. They told me I can go home. They gave me a note for my job, told me to take off for

74

four weeks. They wanted me to focus on me. When I came home, my car was fixed. I found me a place to live, God came through for me. I had a praying mother who always pray for me when I could not. Thank God for a praying mother. I began to dust myself off and start back over, I was back smiling again.

One day I ran across a friend name Carl. I saw him at the store. We knew each other because our parents were best friends. I gave Carl my number and he calls me. One day, I was talking to him over the phone. I ended up telling him we can hook up. I decided to go pick him up. He would cook dinner for me and my kids. He also volunteers to watch my kids, while I go to work. I already had my cousin Tiffany watching my boys, while I work. Carl just wanted to get away from his mother house. I did not want this guy moving in with me. Like I said, I just like his company. Later we became couples, he ended up moving in with me. I wish I never did that. His car was not running, plus he is living with his mother. I got tired of dealing with guys not having their own place. All Carl was good for, was watching my boys and keeping the house clean. Everything else was a poor excuse for a man. When we broke up it did not end well. I always told him if I find someone, they will be bringing more to the table. Patrick started coming back around when he smells a man. One day Carl was using my car. Patrick calls me going off saying, I saw that coward in your car with another woman. Like he never did that himself. I blew it off, and I did mention to Carl what Patrick said. Patrick also had a problem with Carl to. He truly did not like him. Carl did not like him. One night Patrick pops over my house beating on my window. He was screaming my name outside the window. I looked into his eyes, while he looked me into mines. I saw nothing but terror. He did not look the same. Patrick will get where, when things was not running well with his females, he will come and ruin my life. Meanwhile, I had Carl over, I told Carl to hide. Carl hid behind the shower curtains. Patrick start knocking on the door screaming, He want to see his boys. It was 2:30 AM in the morning, here I am dealing with Patrick. I told him to leave from the door. The boys were sleep. He was not listening, he just wanted to scare the hell out of me. I just wanted him to stop bothering me. Patrick ideal was to keep controlling my life. Here I am falling in love with guys that have pass trauma. He used to tell me, I got you before I had kids.

Meanwhile, I reach out to my mom, she will always talk to me about coming back to church. Anytime I have issues, she would tell me to read the word. I did not want to listen; I just wanted her help.

She was trying to send me to God for help. In the beginning, I did not understand it. I completely stop calling her. I did not want to hear about God. I felt like God was mad at me. Later I ended up meeting a married man name Deloria. Deloria treated me like first class. He was smart and intelligent. He always took care of me. I knew this guy was married; I did not care. I knew what I wanted, so I went for it. While dated this married guy, he became jealous. Later I found out, he was an undercover narcissistic. He was good at cheating on his wife. I was not his first. I am glad I ended it with him. I truly felt bad for messing around with this lady husband. No matter how good his money was. Tip, never sleep around with another woman husband.

One afternoon I visited my uncle Anderson. He is my best uncle in the world. Everybody loves

Anderson. One day he told me about this guy name Silos. Uncle told me how cool of a guy he was. Anderson was always saying people are cool. He knew I did not like hanging around his begging friends, he said Silos was not like that. When I met Silos, he was a good guy to talk to. I liked him as a friend. He was someone I can trust. At that time, I had Carl living with me, when I met Silos. I was not feeling Karl anymore. He had shown me how cruel he is. He knew I was getting tired of him and his daughter. Meanwhile, Silos will always take care of my car. We look out for one another. I finally got Carl out my house. I did notice, when I start hanging around Silos, he would go out the way trying to please me. He never told me he liked me, but it showed. As time passed, I start invited him to my house. He would hang around all day. I will feed him and let him shower. We never slept around, He gave me respect. I remember, I got pull over by the police officer. They gave me a ticket

for court. The ticket dated for Sunday. One afternoon, I get a knock at the door. The officer came
to my house and said, they have a warrant on me.
The officer dropped my boys off at my auntie
house. She stayed five minutes away. I was
ashamed that my boys saw me going to jail. This
was my first time in jail. I got release the next day.
Finally, when I went to court. I told the judge, the
officer set my date on a Sunday. The judge said you
should have gotten someone else. I thought I was
going to win this case. I had proof I was in the hospital. That did not matter to them. As time went by,
Silos took me to meet his parents. I Met his father
and Mother. They were nice people that welcome
me in their home with love. Silos was 45 when I
met him. We became close as time went by. I remember one day I was in a situation, that I had to
move. I did not want to move in with Patrick. So, I
moved to Mississippi where Silos Mom had lived.
I lived there for three months. My car was not

running. So, Patrick let me use his car, because he thought I was going to be back with him. I lost feelings for Patrick.

Chapter 7

Meanwhile while moving in with Silos. I never stayed with a man. I will go over Patrick's mother house when Silos made me mad. My boys stayed with their grandma on weekends. I was so stressful about my living situation. Patrick was no help at all. I stopped asking him for his money. Patrick knew when that stop, he had no power over me. As time goes by, I moved out of Silos place and found me my own spot. Silos helped me move my things back to Memphis. I had Silos over my house all the time. I knew this guy was a good man. Later, the job I had; I was not getting enough hours. So, I decided to ask Silos to move in with me. We never had a title for our relationship. Meanwhile I start reaching out to God. I was in a situation that had me running to God. I thought again moving another man would solve it. I was wrong. I was so empty. I decided to go to church. While I was in church, the word spoke to my spirit, so I decided to join the church. My mother invited me. She was already a member at the Healing Center. She was a mother of the Healing Center. When I joined the church, I saw my mother shouting to God, "Thank you Jesus." The Healing Center was the best thing that happen to me. I truly came out the darkness into the light. I came home and told Silos about us living in sin. I told him about the Healing Center and what I learn. I invited him to go to church with me. He came to church with me and fear what he has heard. He did not come back, so I told him I cannot live in sin. I did feel bad that I move him in, and then had to tell him he had to move out. He was sad. I had no control over what I was trying to do for God. I just knew I wanted to change. I wanted to do what is right. As time goes by, me and my boys continue going to church, and bible class. I needed this love; I was looking for the Healing Center. The people there had a beautiful spirit. Everyone there was so nice and caring. Never experienced this inside a kingdom. Later Silos decided to come back to church with me. He came back wanted to be with me. I do not know for sure if he was during it for God. I just felt good I had people in my circle going to church. I told people about my church. I wanted them to feel what I was feeling. Silos join the church, him, and my boys. I was excited that he did that. Later Silos was talking about marriage. Silos said he asked the Lord for a wife. He never said who. I thought that was great. Never thought that he was talking about me. Silos and I continued going to church as a family. One day this lady at my church asked me was I married to Silos. I told her No. She asks me do you all lived together. I said a little bit. So, she started saying if he can live with you, he can marry you. I told her I am not ready. She kept going at me until we got married. Finally, I decided to get married. It was four of us that got married at the same time. I know when we first decided we was going to do it. I was not sure if I should do this. My mother was saying you have boys, they need a father figure. My mother will always say you have to show respect around your boys. This was my first marriage. Finally, Silos found us a house. My kids had their own back yard. I owe this to God. We were finally a family. We put God first in our life. A family that prays together stays together. I always believe in that.

As time went by, I was feeling a little sick, something was going on with my joints. I would always be in pain. I did not know what was going on. My primary doctor said that my face had a butterfly rash. That was a sign of lupus. She gave me an appointment to see the specialist. They assessed my skin. They also gave me medicine to take.

Later they gave me a call to get my test results. I call my uncle to ride with me. I did not want to be by myself. When I get there, the doctor explained to me what they saw. They continued to explain to me about this unknown disease. I had no clue what that was. Nobody I knew had lupus. The doctor told me you could not get rid of this disease. I felt so bad hearing that I had a disease that cannot be cure. When I finally heard someone knew about it. I was speechless. I finally decided to google this illness. An inflammatory disease caused when the immune system attacks its own tissues. Lupus (SLE) can affect the joints, skin, kidneys, blood cells, brain, heart, and lungs. Treatment can help, but this condition cannot. I continued to take my medication and learned more about lupus and how to take care of my skin. I asked the doctor what I must do to make my skin better. He said quit smoking and no red meat. I quit smoking cigarette. I wanted to look better and feel better. Stop smoking truly had helped my skin. My husband was great support. Meanwhile me and the family was loving our new place. The boys love the new school they was going to. We all was going to church as a family. Things was looking good for all of us.

Silos was still taken care of the bills while I wasn't able to work. I was not getting any income at this time because I had Lupus. I didn't know that I can get my social security until later. We got behind in bills because my husband Silos was the only one with income. We slowly stop going to church. Things start to get hard on us all. Until one day we went to court and had to move.

I found us a place to stay when we got our income tax and we paid the rent up for six months. We had to because of our credit was bad. When we move we all went back to church all but my husband. When that started I slow down myself.

My boys was upset that we move to another location. They wanted to stay at the school they was attending. They all were well known in school. The teacher admire my boys strength and obedience.

Finally they started to like the new school they was going to. My son Tevin was in the band for many years. My youngest son Cortez play football. He was good at it.

My oldest son Jeffrey was known as well. All the girls love him.

My son Tevin made good grades all through the school year and graduated with honors.

My three boys truly made me a proud mom until one day I got a call.

My oldest son Died in a bad car wreck. I get a knock on the door and it was his cousin Terrence. He was shaking and nervous. I knew something was wrong because it was after 12PM. He said Peaches Patrick died in a bad car wreck. My heart stop and I was trying to make sure I was hearing this right. He repeated it again. He broke down and cried trying to explain what had happened. I didn't have any words. My husband was trying to get me to respond or say something. My husband start saying maybe he is April fooling us. Because my son died on That day. I knew terrence wasn't playing with me. Terence left and I call the police station to see what is going on. They did not tell me anything. They said if anything happened to your son someone will come to your house. I waited for hours to see if my son died. The feeling of trying see if your son died felt heavy on my heart. I wasn't able to breathe correctly. I call again to see will someone tell me something. I didn't get anything. I try to call him to see will he answer his phone.

Finally I saw lights outside my window. My husband said the police are outside. Lord knows I wasn't myself at that moment. They knock on the door and my husband answer the door. They ask for Angela Fitts I came to the door. They ask me for some ID. I present it to them. As I show them it was three officer. One said I'm sorry to say your son Patrick Moten Died in a bad car wreck. Him and his cousin Whom were with him. He continued to say they died instantly without suffering.

While he was explaining this to me. I wasn't able to breathe at this point. I realized I was having a panic attack. At that moment I thought I Half Died. I wanted the officer to stop talking. I remember asking them Why didn't nobody come get me. My son died alone. I wasn't there for him. I was screaming that to the officers. They was saying that they are gone. They move the body. I was so done at that moment. I ask them to please leave let me be. They said ok I'm sorry this happened .

I remember my husband put his arms around me and held me said I'm here. My body was so none and sore. My eyes was full of tears and pain. I felt that pain through my soul. God knew I wanted to give up.

I finally call my Mother to explain to her that her grandson died. When she answer I remember saying Mom Patrick died in a bad car wreck. I was trying to breathe as I was explaining this to her.

She wasn't able to respond. I continue to explain to her what I knew and the tears started to drown me as I continue to talk. Meanwhile My Step-Dad Willie got the phone and He was asking what was wrong. I explain to him the best I could. The more I try to express myself I noticed I was steady panic and trying to breathe. I remember Dad saying do you need us to come over. I told him not right now because I wanted to finish crying. I was just hoped I was going to wake up and this was going to be a dream. The pain was so hard to carried.

I later got in touch with my other two boys. They stay overnight with some friends. When they came home I explain to them the best I could. It was so hard trying to tell my boys there brother died. I didn't not want them to see me cry or see my pain. I did all I can to hide it from them. When I told them. I knew that it would hurt there little soul. I did not want my boys to experience so much pain. Watching my boys hurt broke me down into small pieces.

I remember so many people praying for us and trying to uplift me. I was so none. I did not feel anything. I did not have any fight in me. I was so happy we had Life Insurance. That helps a lot when your mind is not there. I know someone was praying for me to give me strength to buried my son. That was the hardest thing a mom can do. We had his cousin buried with him. Remember they both died together. My son was the driver. They was speeding and lost control of the car.

Hearing that my son was speeding broke my spirit. I start thinking it was my fault because I should have told him to be careful more. I also thought like if me and his father never got him a car he would still be here. I punished myself for a long time about his death. My behavior start to change. I noticed I was becoming someone else I didn't like.

I became so depressed about losing my son. I hated a lot of things. I remember people I see will look just like him. I will ride down the street thinking I saw my son. Life was so hard. My Lupus has got the best of me. I was in a mission with my sickness. I wasn't taken care of myself like I should. I was died slowly on the inside.

I completely stop going to church. I shut down from my husband. I noticed I start gaining weight. I continue trying to live without my son. My other two boys became known at there school. They was doing good in school. Nothing bad was going on with us. I was keeping my pain to myself. I wanted the best for my boys.

I watch them go to school and make a life for themselves. I was so proud of them. That made me happy again. I was coming alive until Tevin left home to go to college. I was so afraid to see him leave. My anxiety started kicking in bad. I had to start walking so I can clear my mind from these negative thoughts. I still had my youngest son at home with me. I was proud of him as well. When he graduated high school and got himself a car he move out.

Now it just me and my husband Silos. I'm trying make our house a home without my boys. I start having these negative thoughts that will come and go. This time it lead me to a guy name Willie. I met Willie on facebook. I friend request him because I knew him years ago. I finally decided to say something to him. He responded fast. He ask me to come over his house so he can see who I am. I felt like I should.

I wanted to take my mind off what I had going on in my life. When he told me he had his own place. I said great because most mens I met never did. Plus I wanted to be in another atmosphere. As I talk to him about coming to his house. I was so nervous because I really didn't know what I was getting myself into. I said to myself he can be a good friend to talk to.

As I went to his place he was already outside and it was hot. I pull up to his place and roll my window down ask for him. As he was approached my car. I was saying to myself he do not look like the guy in the picture. He was tall and goofy looking. When He spoke to me I noticed a lot of negative things about him. I ask him while we were sitting in my truck can I use his bathroom. I wanted to see what his place look like. Plus he already was looking like he just woke up.

We came in his house he had two big dogs in a one bedroom house. He did mention he had to go to work that day. That is one reason I came because I knew he had to work. I wanted someone to talk to about my son. I noticed most people got tired of hearing about my son patrick. Having a new person around they want get bored. I decided to be his friend because we had a lot in common.

I stay over his house until he had to go to work. I did tell him I was married. He didn't have a problem with that. What I like about Willie was he was real. Willie made it very easy for me to be his friend. He would always text nice things I like to hear. I still was hurt about losing my son as I continue to conversation with this guy. After I left his house we made plains to see each other again. I told him Friday. He call and said come see him he cannot wait until Friday.

I came over his house sat with him until my husband got off from work. That day I knew I was going to love hanging out with him. As time go by we started to get closer. He ask me will I put my name on his light bill. I hardly knew him to be doing things like that. He ask me to come over, I came and his lights was off. He would turn them off during the day. Have the lights on at night. That means he was using MLGW lights without permission. Here I am saving the day. I decided to go ahead and put my name on his light bill. I ask him who name was it in at first. He try to brush it off by saying they didn't pay there light bill. Willie said I need someone who is responsible to pay bills so he want get his light cut off. So MLGW connected it through my account. Remember I ignored the red flag. Willie needed help paying bills. He couldn't pay his rent and light bill without been behind. He also start half paying on it. That is when I step in and start paying the light bill myself to keep my credit good. He said it was only temporary. Then we start playing house. Willie was treated me like his main chic. He wanted me around all the time. I truly forgot about the pain I was going through with my son.

I began to start falling for this guy. I wasn't coming home until it was time to take my husband to work. Silos didn't question anything I do. I was kinda piss because Willie will say my husband must be seeing someone else. I knew my husband wasn't seeing nobody. He wanted me to think bad things about my husband. That right there is a red flag speaking down on my husband. I continue to ignore his red flags because I knew I was in the dark. I didn't want anyone to see me. I did know what I was doing was wrong. I just didn't want to face the pain.

I was willing to do anything to not think about my son or been at home in a unhappy home. Meanwhile Willie couldn't keep him a job at all. His mouth will get him in trouble. He would have to find work somewhere else. It didn't take him long to find work. One day Willie decided to move. He made me feel like you are the woman of the house. I transferred the lights over to his new place. Things was beginning to look good for him. Until he lost his job again.

He ended up working with his father in Jackson Mississippi. He will come home for the weekend. He gave me a key to his place to keep an eye on his place and his dog. I became close with his dog.

I took good care of his place while he was away. I took care of my place and his. I did a good job at it. In the beginning I thought it was fun having two guys that care about me. I had to find out the hard way karma was around the corner waited for me.

Willie treated me good when he was working out of town. When he lost his job with his dad. He changed again. That mask was off for good. He show me who he really was. He came home and found him another job. When he got on his feet he wanted to start seeing other females. So he ask for his key back. When he ask for his key, I stop helped him pay bills. He didn't know I was going to do that. He began to act funny with me. He started telling me to call before I come. He start putting rules down for me. I got mad.

Willie already knew I fell for him and he started acting differently. The text stop coming. I decided to cut the lights off. I told him I was going to do it. He didn't believe me because I always threat him I would. Finally I decided to cut them off. I knew that it would break up things with us. I started to feel that he was using me for anything I had to offer. He was needed. Every time i see him he need things. When I cut the lights off. I call him and told him.. He also left an outstanding balance that i had to pay. I did feel bad about it. I knew this was the best thing to do. He was very disappointed and hurt. When Willie ghosted me, I lost it! I did not understand how this guy could just up and block me. I wanted to get revenge on him. I wanted him to feel my pain. I distance myself from family and friends. I did not want anyone to know he hurt me. I remember, I was afraid to go to sleep at nights. My anxiety was bad. I did not trust anyone or anybody. I wanted to destroy this guy for what he did to me.

I end up reaching out to another guy named Raheem. He was a soldier. I met him on Facebook. He added me on his Facebook. I always thought he was nice looking. Never said anything to him until Willie hurt me. I decided to meet up with him. It was a nice and pretty day. I told him to meet me at the park. We liked each other on the spot. We could not wait to see each other again. He would text me all during the day. In the beginning he was moving too fast for me. He wanted me to come over every day. I could not, because I had a husband. I just wanted to stop thinking about Willie. I later found out that Raheem is a narcissistic as well. I almost started to fall for this guy. He told me things I like hearing. We only dated months. It did not last long. He turns me off when he started asking me for money. He could never keep a job or a steady income. I said to myself, he is just like Willie. I told him about Willie. That was the wrong thing to do. He uses that against me. He was a little jealous about me been married and having Willie. He was a special narcissistic.

Oh, I forgot to mention Willie and I got into it about this female calling him. He was asleep. I answer his phone. I knew who she was. I saw the name come across the phone. She asks for him, and I told her no. Knowing that I was married. I did not care. I woke him up mad. He did not know what was going on till, I gave him his phone and left. He jumped in his truck and followed me home. Willie was yelling pull over, I did not. He was calling me; I would not answer his calls. He continued to follow me to my house. I turned down another street. He pulled up at my house blowing his horn. He knew my husband was in the house. My husband came out the house. Willie was screaming telling him to tell your wife to stay away from his house. I never thought Willie will have done anything like that. I did not know why he would tell my husband about us. He waited for me to call him. I just could not get past how he would do me like that. I knew this guy had an evil spirit that would kill steal and destroy. I remembered my husband saying, Willie cannot have his wife.

One summer, I was having problems with my heart. I went to the doctor, and they gave me a physical examination. I was told two days later I had a silent heart attack. I did not take it seriously. I continue to ignore the signs. I was dealing with mixed emotions. I was afraid to face my situation. I start having panic attacks. I was losing control over everything. I was always having flares in my body. One day, I was having bad chest pain. I thought it was gas or maybe chest pain. I continue with my daily life. Until one day, I could not take the pain. I told my husband how hard it was to eat. The pain was tense. I told my husband to take me to the emergency hospital. When I got there, they ran a test on me. The doctor said they had to keep me for procedure. I called my mother and told her what was going on. I told her everything was okay. Later, I told my husband to go to work. I was thinking they had to run more test. I had no idea they were going to have surgery. They prepared me up for surgery. After all this was over, they brought me back to recover. They explained to me what they did. I was not able to walk or move my arm. They placed a stent in my heart. The stent allowed blood to flow through the previously blocked artery. After having my surgery, I had to start back over. I had to go to rehab for eight weeks. They had to check my heart. I made sure I did my eight weeks. I got a certificate for attending.

After I finished rehabilitation, I joined a gym. Dac is the name of the gym. I took care of my health and my well-being. I was determined to fight. I was going to the gym daily. I met people at the gym. The first lady I start talking to was Gwen. We always did fun things together besides the gym. We went to the zoo, out to eat, movie and shopping. I invited her to my church. She has a good heart. People like Gwen, you will want to keep around. I met this lady name Sabrina. She is an instructor for the gym. I met her at the pool. Sabrina approaches me and asked me will I like to join her classes in the pool. I was so happy she asked me. I smiled and said sure. Sebrina treated me like a mom. She and I pray together. I met so many nice people in the pool. Sabrina and I will do lunch and bible class. The gym was my second home. I also met instructor name Lashawnda. Lashawnda teaches Zumba class. She has this shine when she dances. I have respect for her. I love dancing with Lashawnda. I love when Lashawnda tells me I can do it. I have grown to love her. There is one more instructor I am crazy about. Her name is Cyrilla. Cyrilla classes is tense. I take majority of her classes. Cyrilla shows you how to work out correctly. She has patience for me. That is one reason I love her.

Chapter 8

Meanwhile, I was still attending church. I start been a greeter at my church. I felt good about this. I belong to the Healing Center Baptist Church. I love my church. It changes my life. I respect My Bishop and Pastor Diana Young. I care for all the members inside the church. I met this lady named Gloria and Loraine at the Healing Center. These two ladies were special to me. We minister together. I remain friends with Gloria. These two are my sisters in Christ. Gloria and I have grown close. Gloria is just like a sister to me. I can always be me around her. My pastor Diana is first lady at the healing center. She is a bold and intelligent woman of God. I genuinely appreciate her. Pastor and bishop loves their members. Everyone there show respect to one another. We are a family at the

Healing Center. I thank God for this church. I would not be where I am at now if it were not for the Healing Center Prayers. I been going there over 21 years. My church teaches you about the bible. That is one thing I love about my church. They do not judge. Meanwhile as I am healing from losing my son. I was trying to find something to keep my mind on God. God was talking to me. He has my attention. I was building a relationship with God. He wanted me to let it go. I was having a tough time trying to understand. The Lord put his arms around me and told me he loves me. God forgave me for cheating on my husband. I began to walk with God. I put him first. Everything I did, I wanted to please God. I wanted God to be pleased with me. God asked me to forgive the people that hurt you. I was having a tough time forgiven. I continued to walk with him, but I could not rest until I answer God.

Finally, I was willing to do anything because my anxiety will not turn me lose. I read the bible and pray to God to help me to forgive. He held me in his arms again. I was able to breathe. Letting go of hate made my health better. I was able to be in Gods light. It was a new feeling that God given me. I start praising God for allowing me to do this again. He given me another chance to be happy. When I began to Love Jesus, it was so easy to love people. The Healing Center teaches you that in bible class. One day I decided to open a support group on Facebook. I name the group Psychopathic Narcissist Survivor Support Group. I did this because I wanted to share my story about Narcissistic. I wanted the world to know about these evil people. I knew this would help me. The group began to grow. I pray to God for more followers. Two months later, I open another group on Facebook. How to Live with Anxiety and Panic Behavior. I also suffer with anxiety. I wanted to help people face their fear. The Narcissistic Support Group helped me through my pain, from all the broken relationship I experience. I was able to forgive and let go of that hate and jealous. I saw myself healing. God kept sending more people. I ended up with two platform. I had moderators that was willing to helped me with the group. I was so proud of myself. I work with so many moderators. I needed them more then they know. Later I decided to open a lupus support group. I opened two pages. One is Living with Lupus and How to Live with Lupus. I wanted to help people and share what I go through on a daily basic. I am a warrior, and a mouthpiece for the Lord. We are warriors that battle a sickness that is unknown. I learned to fight so I can live. We get up daily tried to fit in with others. We tell people we are during great just to fit in. I also open another group call, The Broken Relationship/Sisterhood. I thank God for this group as well. I want this group here to be known. This group is a support group. I open this group to help people heal. I want people to learn how to love themselves. The last group I opened is Coming out the darkness. This group helps people break family cycle. Most people grew up in toxic and abused home. I want to help people come out the darkness and share their story. I want people to learn not to be afraid of others. I learned in bible class, we are here to please God not each other. I had to learn that the hard way.

I forgot to mention my friend Sasci. I met her on Facebook. Sasci was not from Memphis. I immediately became friends with Sasci. She and I was going through the same thing. She lost her mom from lupus. She and I support one another. We also were hurt from been in a toxic relationship with the narcissistic. We talk on the phone every day. We always talk about helping people from been with a narcissistic. –Sasci and I grew to love on each other. I can tell her anything. I am so glad she was there to hold my hands. I am grateful that I met her. She will always be a part of my life. She finally, I have not reach out to my kids' father at all. I have been hearing that he has not been doing good. He has been in and out of the hospital. I did reach out to his significant other. She would keep me posted about his situation. I try to respect her and my husband. I did not want to hurt them, by visiting him in the hospital. One morning, my son put on Facebook that is dad had died. I was devastated to hear that my kids' father had died. I at once told my husband. I remember logging off Facebook and the groups. I at once started to blame myself. I had the leaders in the group praying for me. The group held me down. I got on my knees and prayed to God for wisdom. He heard my prayer. I told my boys; they still have their mother. I dust myself off and got back in the groups. I knew I had a mission for the Lord. Prayer is the key. I promise God, I will never run from my position again. God is looking for strong Christians to do his mission. Losing my kids father made me decided to reach out to my dad. He did not answer the call, but he did call back. He sounded down. He explains to me what was going on with him. I at once prayed for him. Melvin said, nobody knew he was sick. He told me to keep this between us. I said OK. He promises me when he gets better, he will call me. I knew he would call me back because he was fighting for his life. He explains to me, he had a virus. I wanted to visit him. I knew that it was not safe to do so. I just kept him in my prayers and waited for his call. As time went by, I heard my cousin mention he ask about me. I told her I talk with him. He promises to call me when he gets better. Shay tries to explain, he still might be going through. Later I saw him on my husband page. He had pictures with his girls. I said well dam. That hit hard. I got frustrated thinking negative thoughts. I decided to pick up the phone and give him a call. As I was calling, he did not answer the call. He called me back and said who is this? I said Peaches your daughter. He is always asking me who is this when I call. He does not know that bothers me. He had the same number for years. Anyway, he gets on the phone with an attitude. Like I have been worried him. He said to me he is not well. He went on saying the doctor said this and that. I got furious again. I am begging him to call me. He did not care or try to explain. He was trying to get off the phone. He never liked to explain himself. I got off the phone crying. I called my mother asking, why he do not talk to me. I know she got tired of me running behind my dad. She prayed for me and told me to let him be. Time went on, I still think about my dad, especially when my kids' father died.

Finally I am in church for good. God has saw fit to give me a chance to live for him. As I look back over my life I came a long way. I pray my story can help someone else. I did this because God ask me to. He brought little me out of a toxic broken relationship and heal me. He also forgiven me for all my sins. He given me a chance to walk with him He will do the same for you if you just let it go and believe. Remember forgive the people that hurting you so you can be happy. Forgive so you want have to live in boundaries. I pray this book will bless someone soul.

I belongs to the Healing Center Baptism Church Bishop William Young And Pastor Diana Young is my pastor. I been going to this church over 20 years. I serve as a greeter. I'm faithful to my church. I'm married to Silos Fitts for 19 years now. He is my king and I'm his Queen. My Mother is Gracy Lewis she is my Queen and my Supporter. She is married to Willie Lewis who is my stepfather for many years. He has held my hand the day He married my mother. My Step-Mother is Pauline Fitts I'm so blessed to have her in my life. My Two boys Cortez Moten and Tevin Moten his wife Nicole Moten.

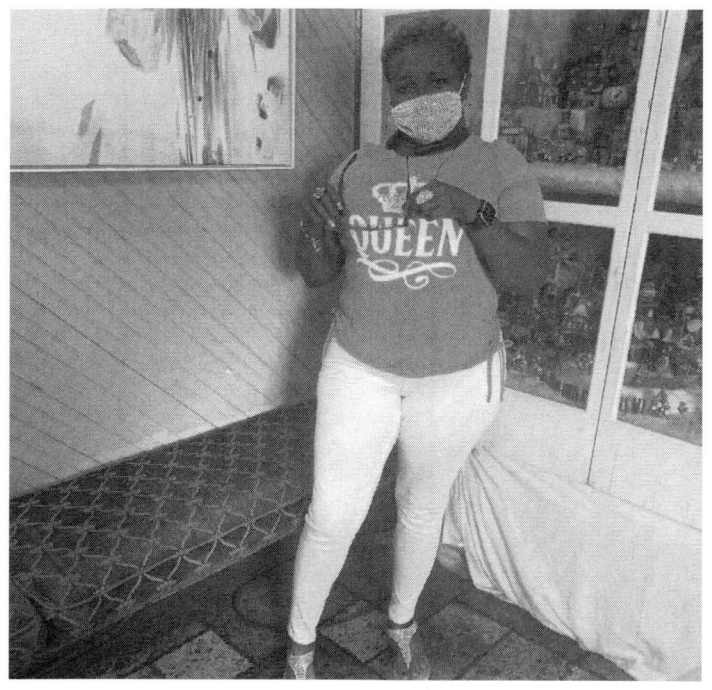

I'm blessed to have these three standing beside me. I thank God for my grandson AJ he brought happiness in my life. Last My only brother Kevin Jordan I did it .

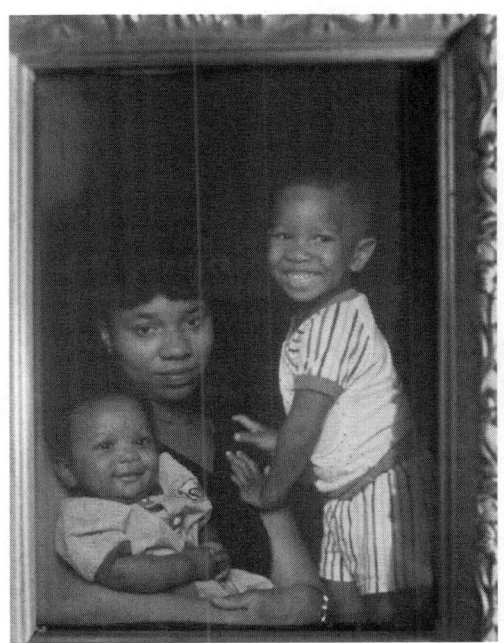

Me and my best friend Yolanda 30 plus years.
Friends forever. We have great memories we share.
We held each other down for many years.
God kept our friendship together.

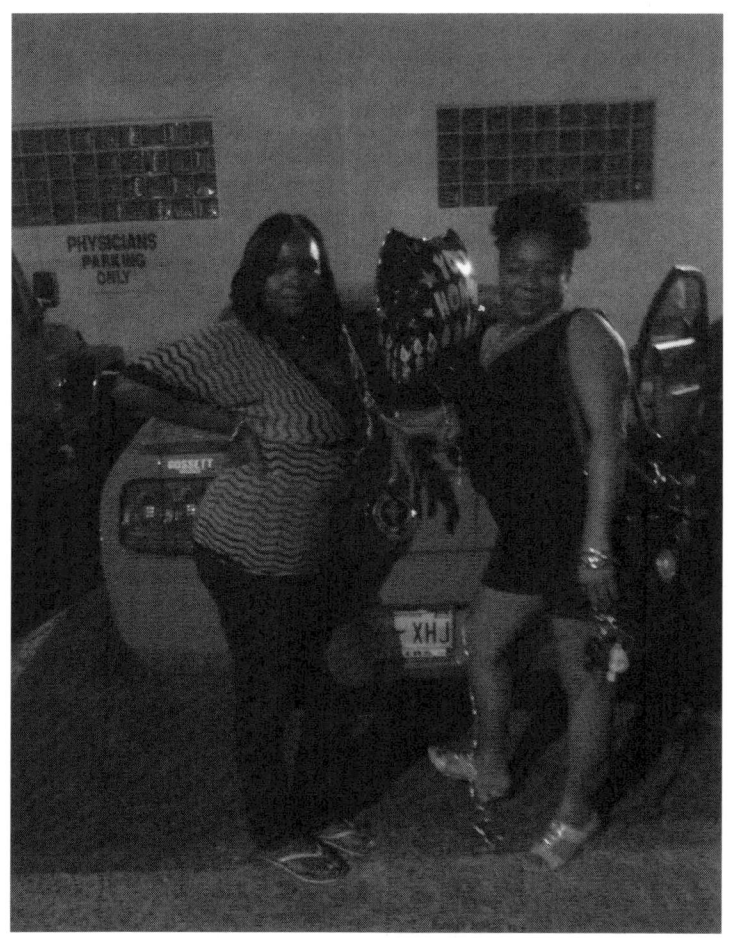

My babies I was so complete.

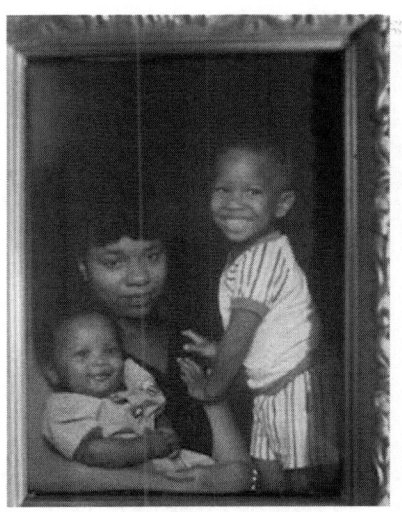

I Am A Warrior I live to be happy and free.

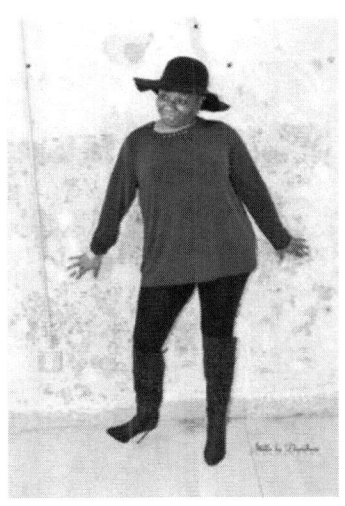

I was 19 Years old. You couldn't tell me anything.
I was sassy and double trouble.

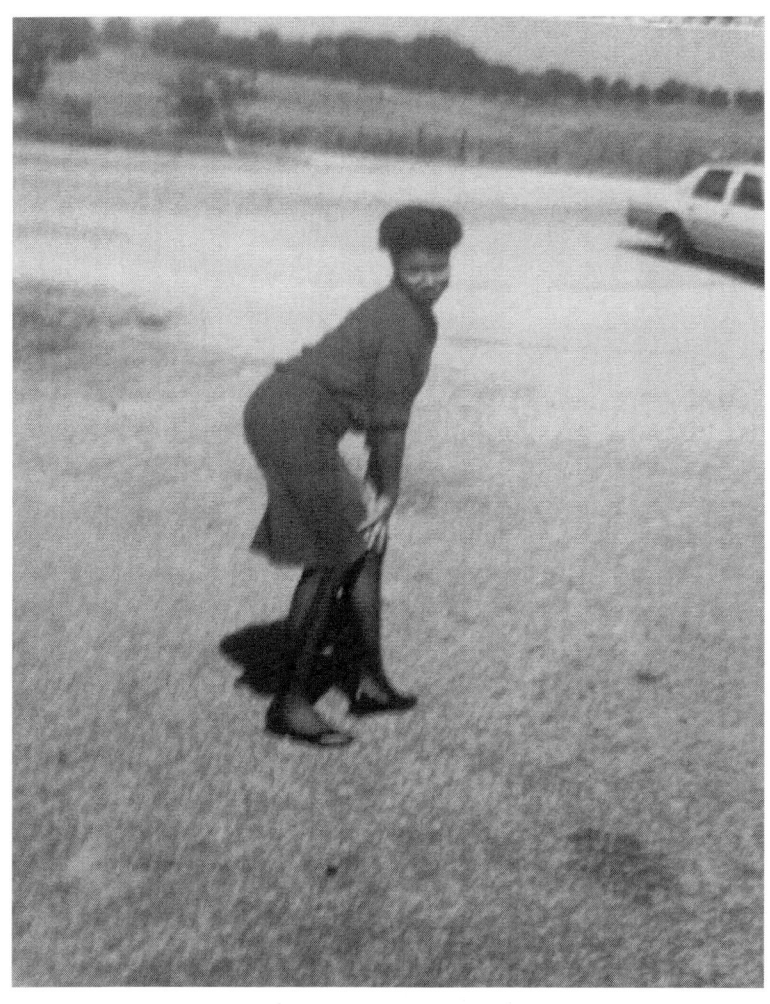

Peaches I never understood why I didn't smile as a child.

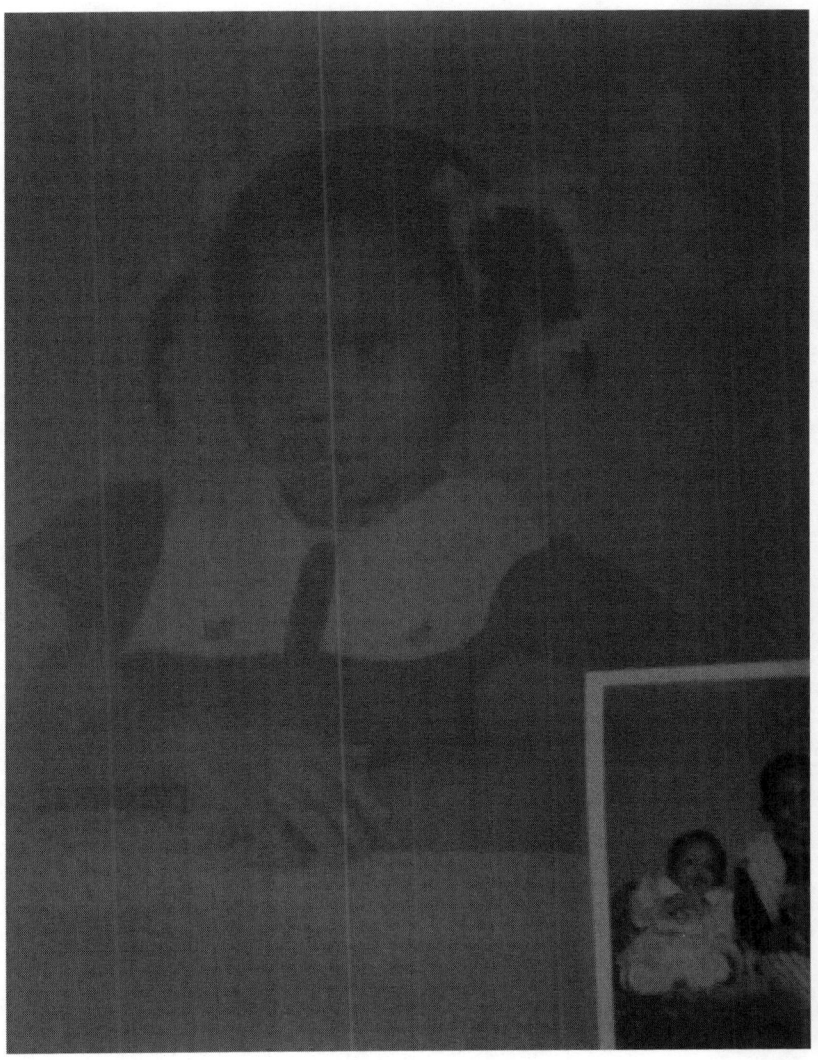

Yes Peaches I was 25 on this picture. Still trying to find myself. I did have my own everything.

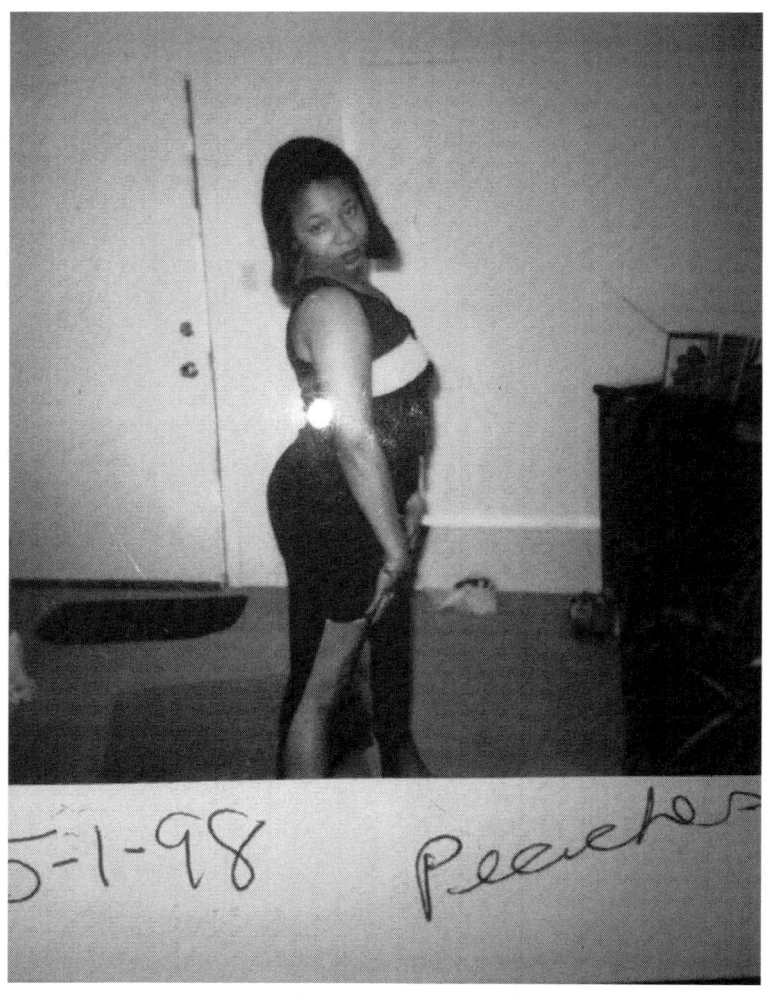

I love me some Peaches.

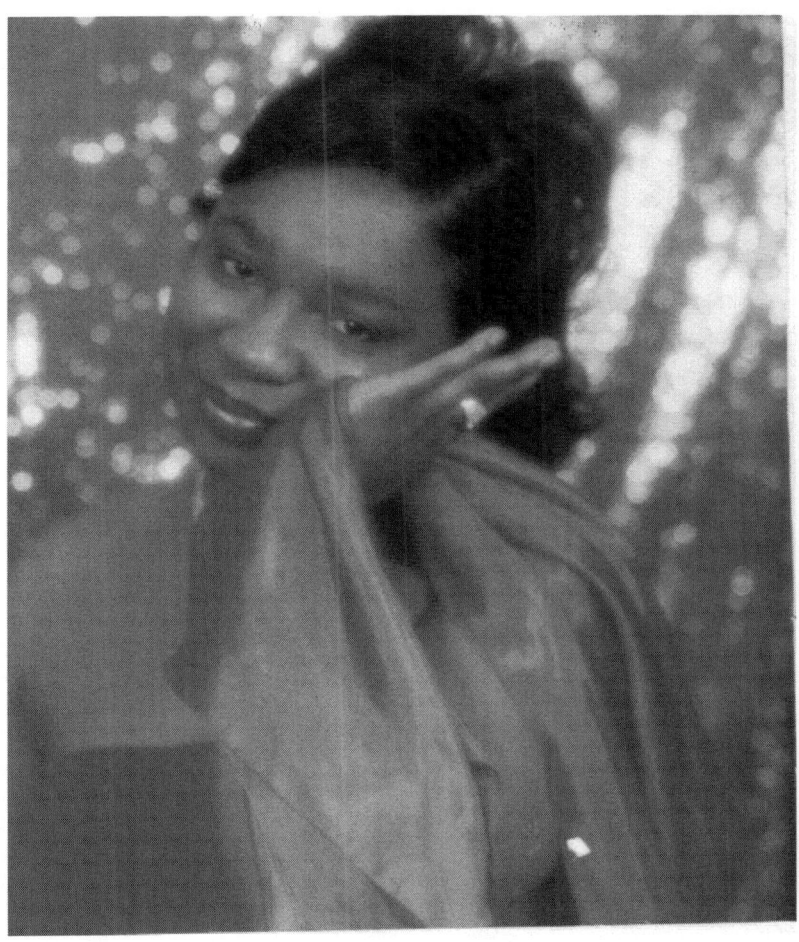

my mother name me peaches she said i was so beautiful.

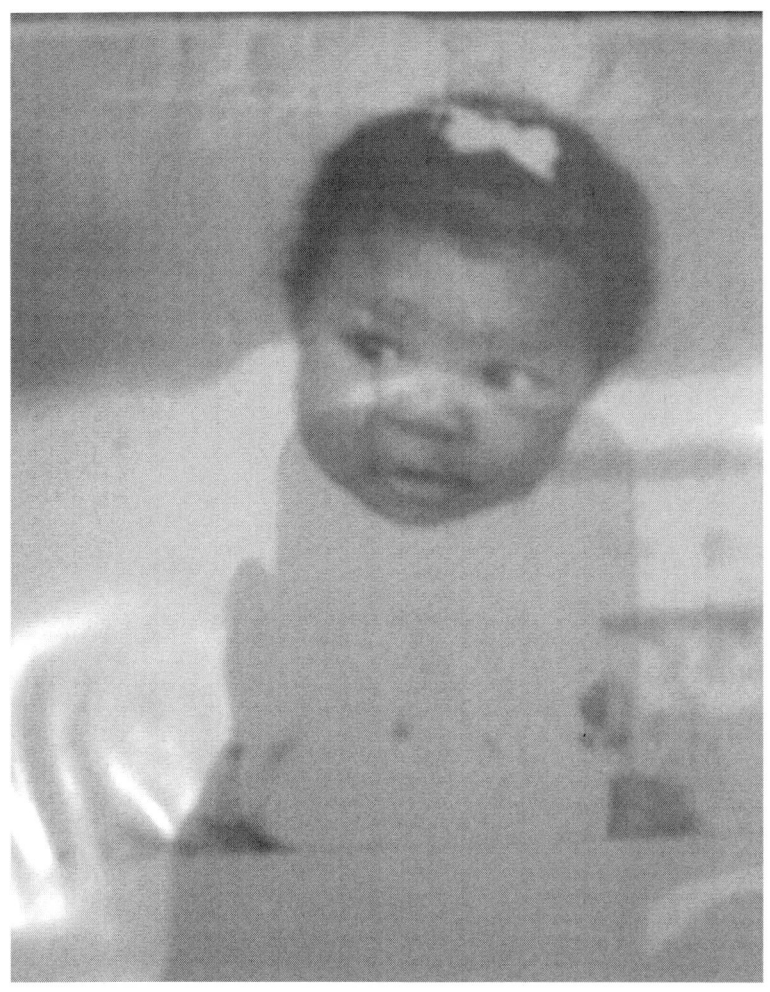

My family my brother and Mother. We were so close we did everything together as a family. Mom kept us in the church and made sure we pray.

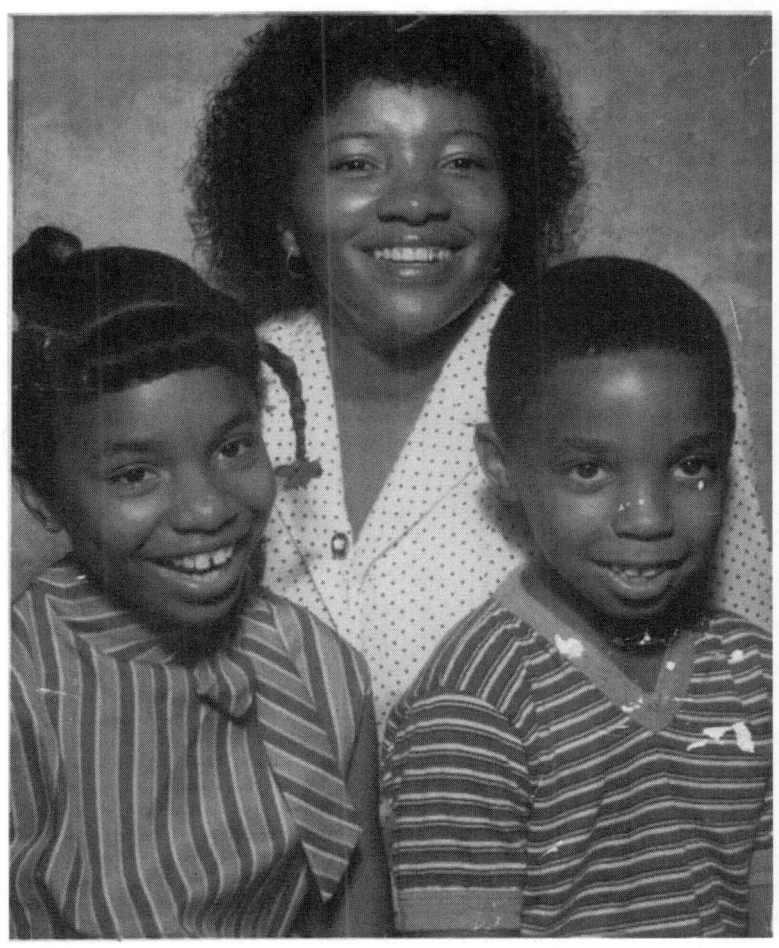

My mother and her first grandson. She was so happy on this day. They actually was happy together.

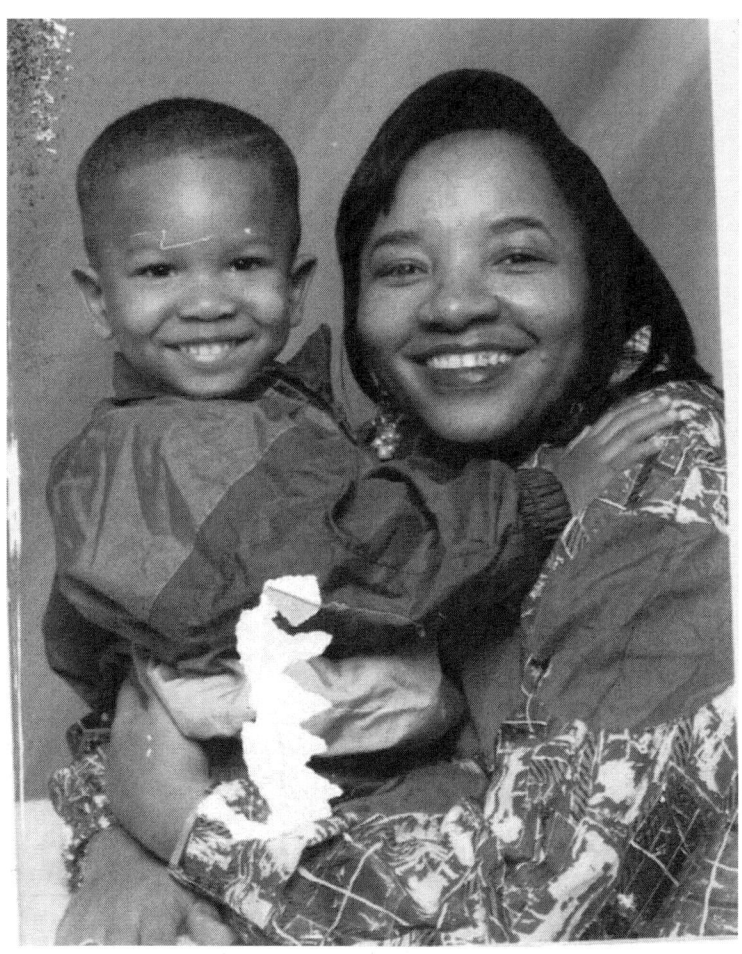

A warrior a survivor a Mother and wife. I believe in Jesus who strength me and gave me a light to shine. I'm forever grateful.

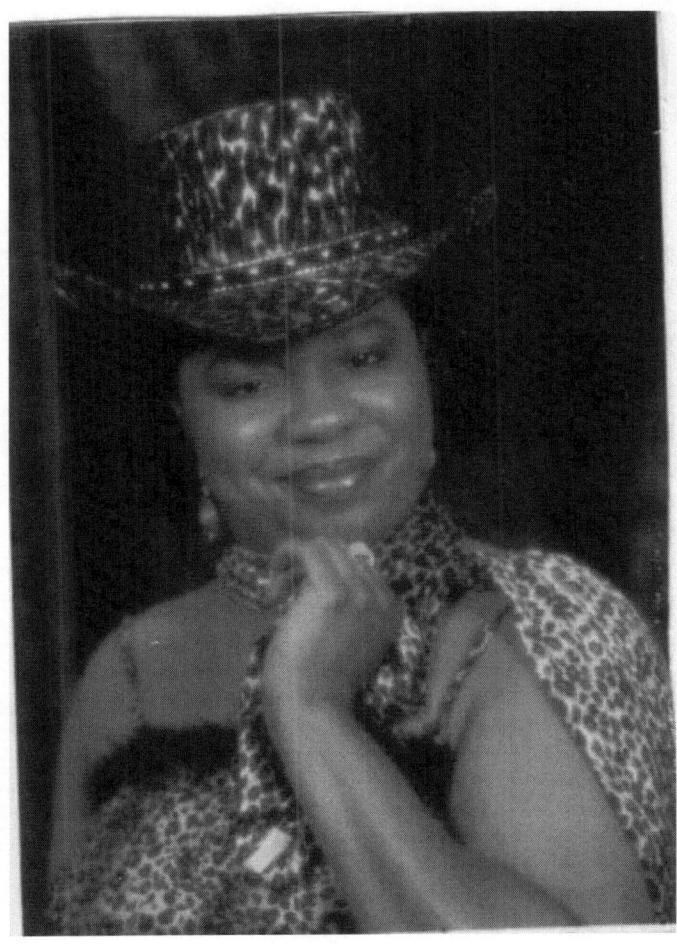

Yes this is me. Smiling like i saw Jesus

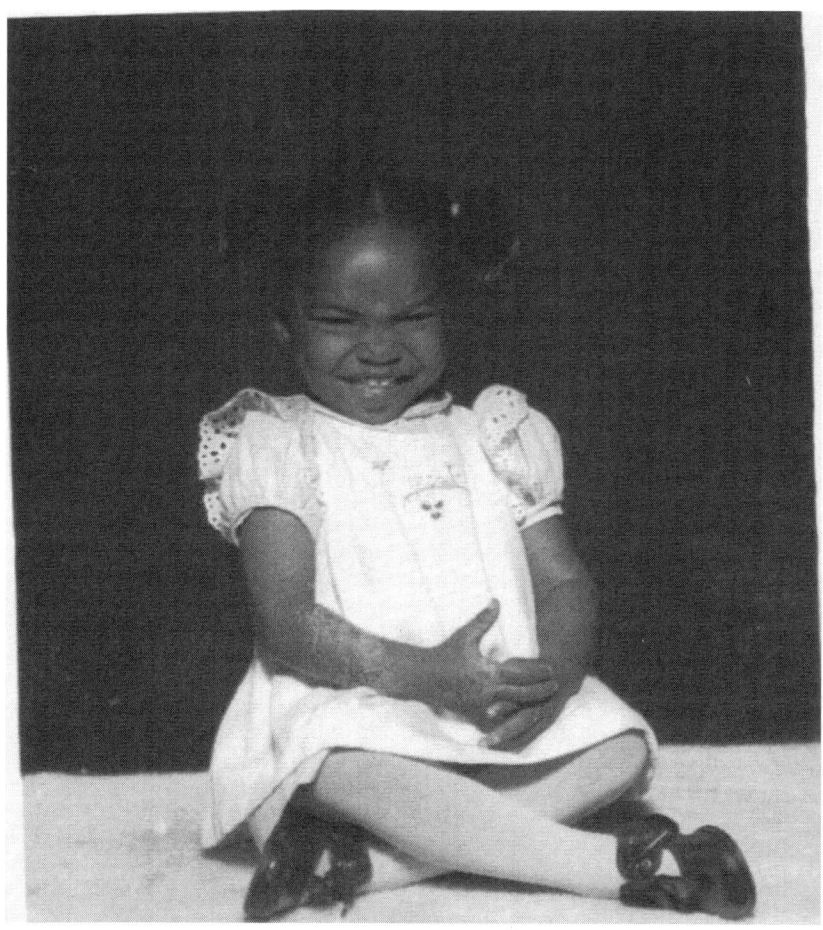

I remember this like it was yesterday. I was 24. This here let's me know I love myself .

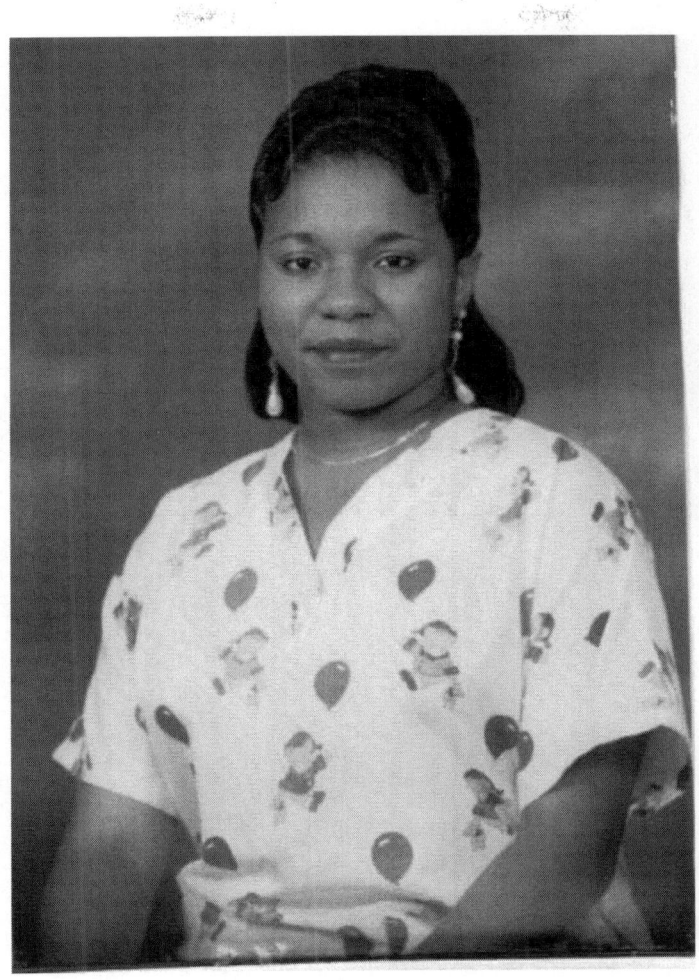

I took this picture on Jeffrey 18 birthday. This is the last time we were together as a family. I cherish this picture.

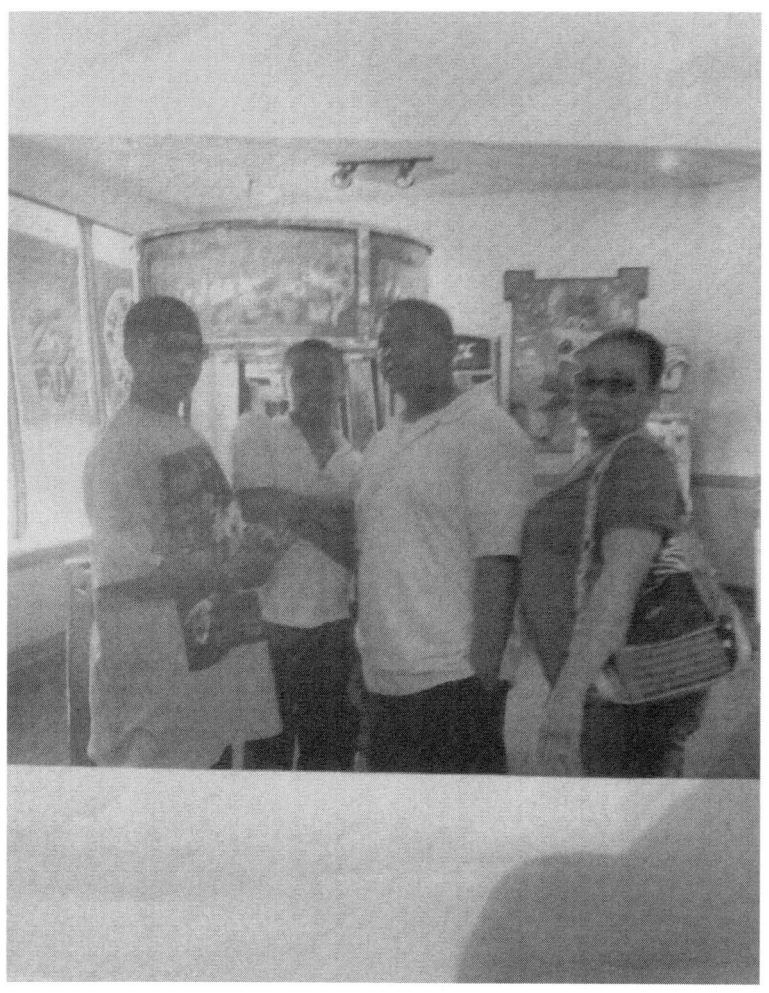

My Three heartbeat. They will do anything to see me happy.

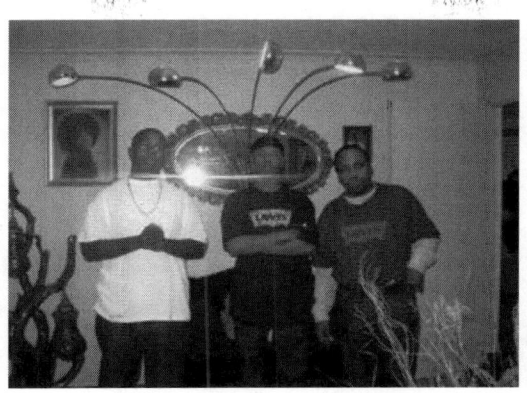

The best thing Jeffrey have me was these three boys. I lived for them.

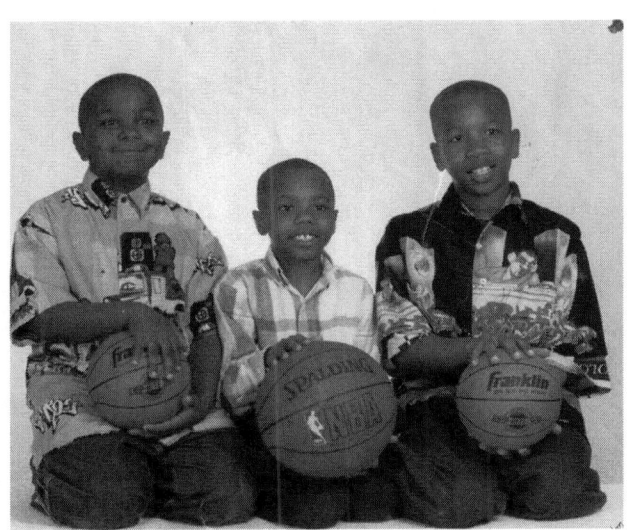

My mother and I. She is my Queen I will
always be my mother keeper.

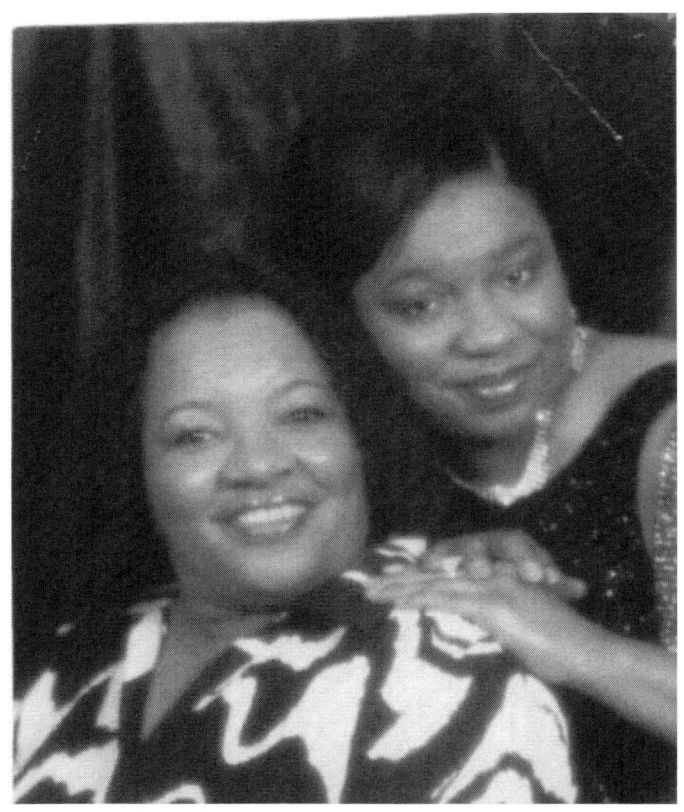

Mrs.Fitts

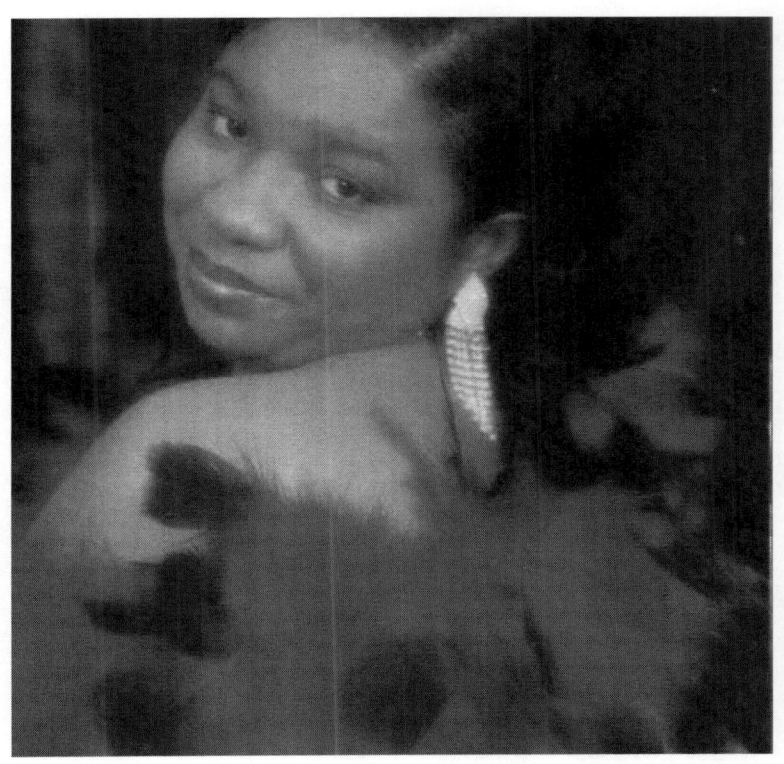

This is the day I had to say goodbye to my oldest son. This is a pain I thought I will never get over. God open up the doors for me and wrap his arms around me show me love.

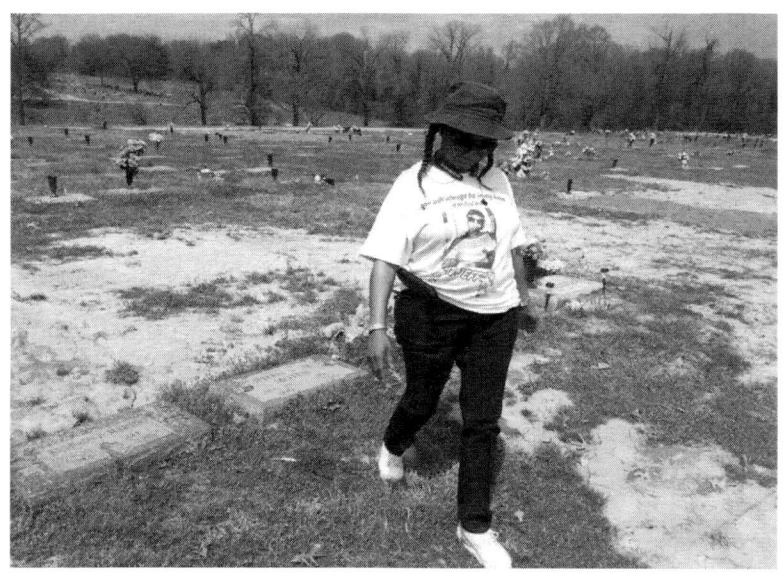

I lived for these two. I'm so grateful to still have them in my life. They truly made me happy and proud mom.

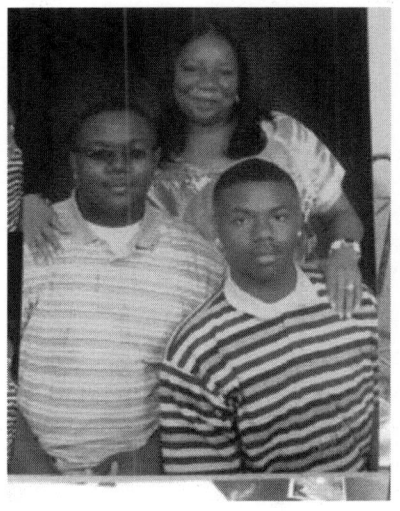